Chronobiology - The Science of Biological Time Structure

Edited by Pavol Svorc

Published in London, United Kingdom

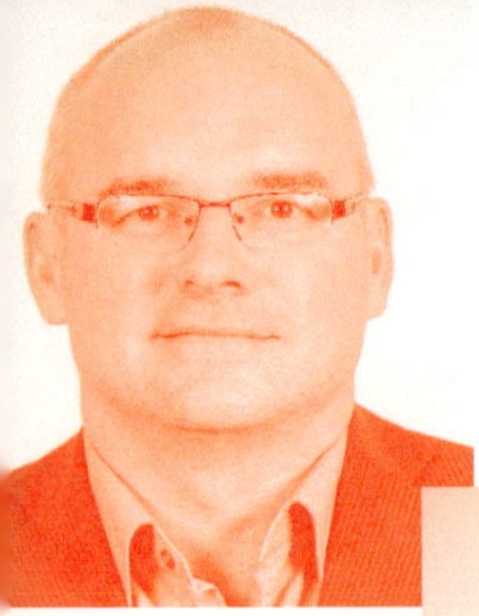
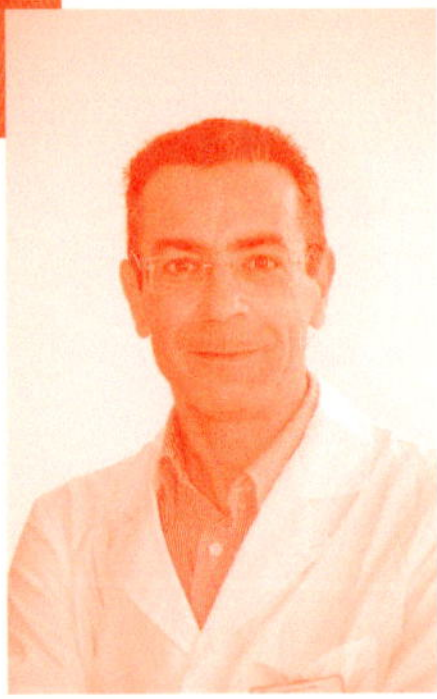
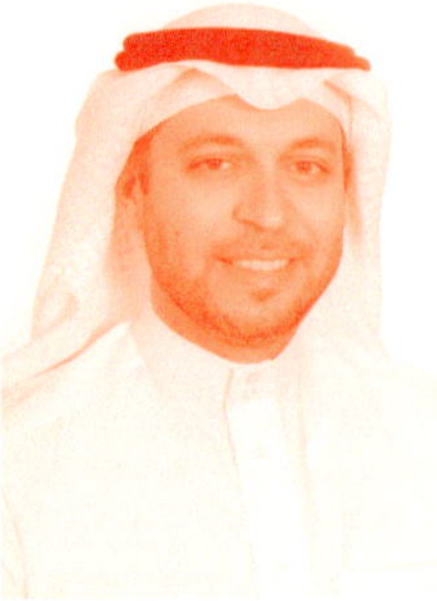
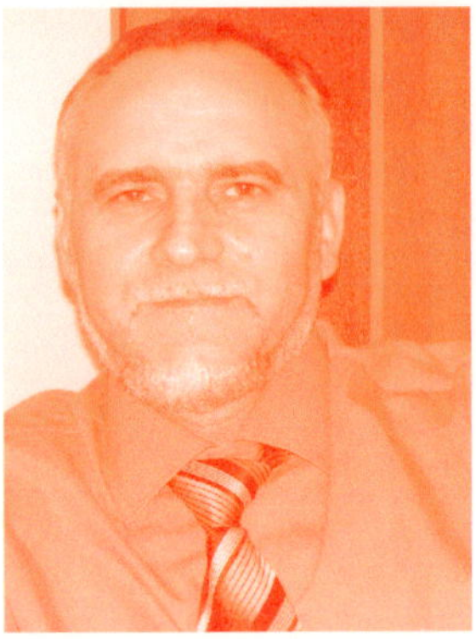
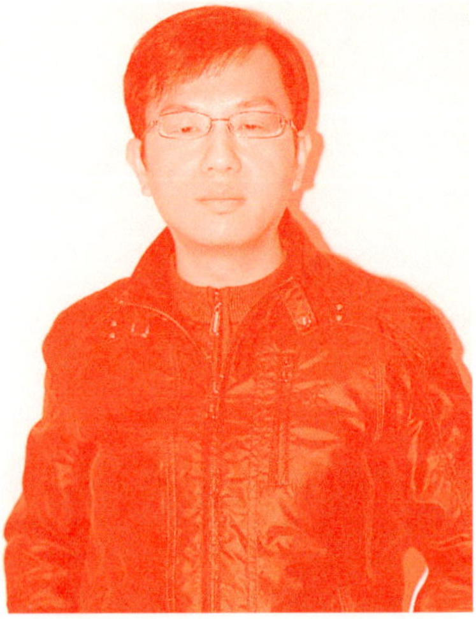
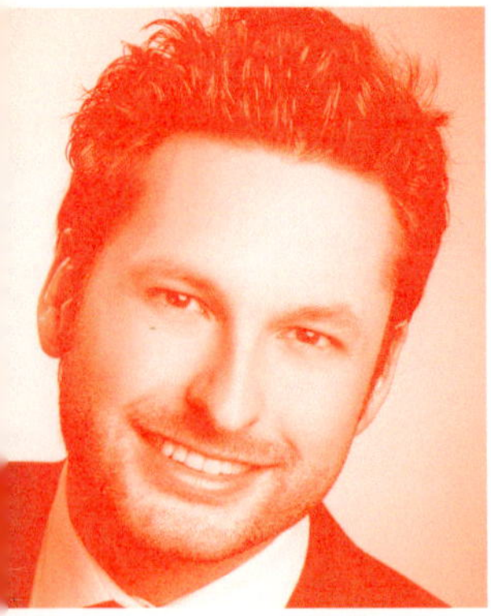
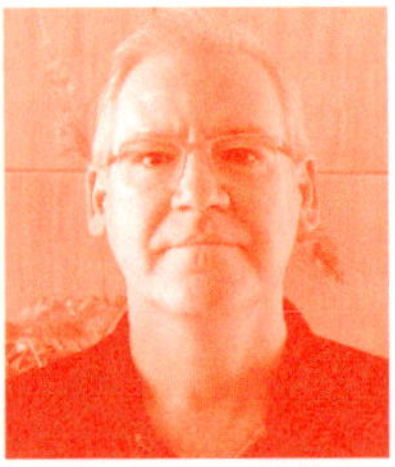

IntechOpen

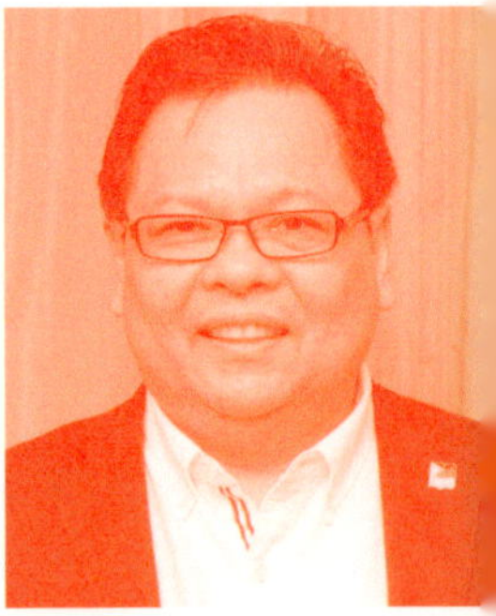
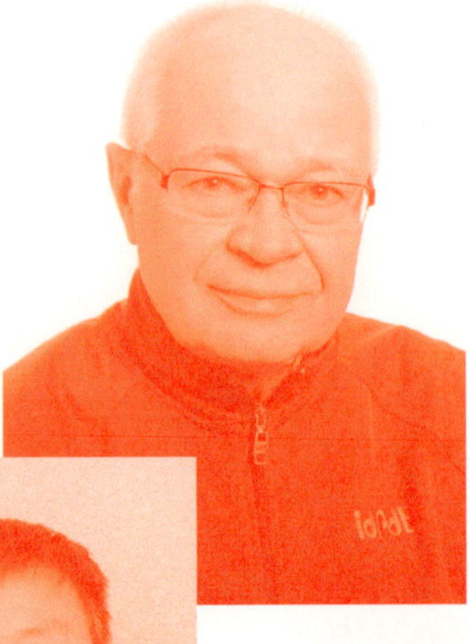
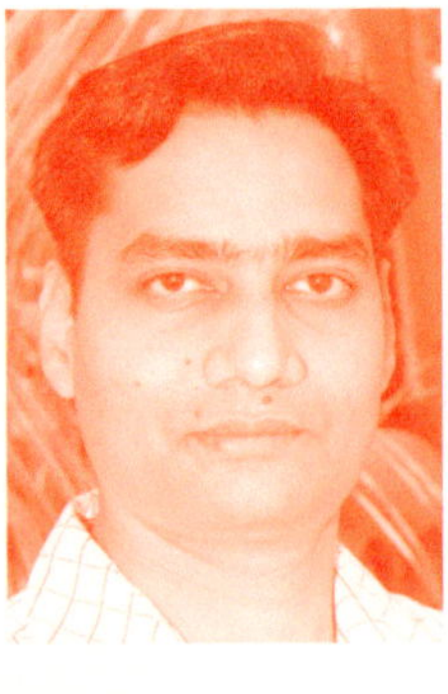
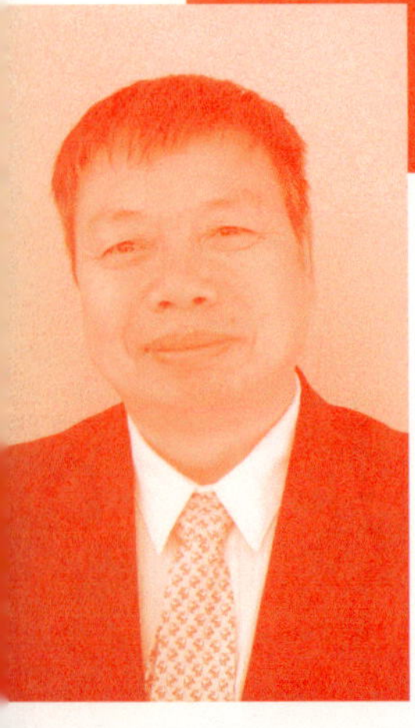
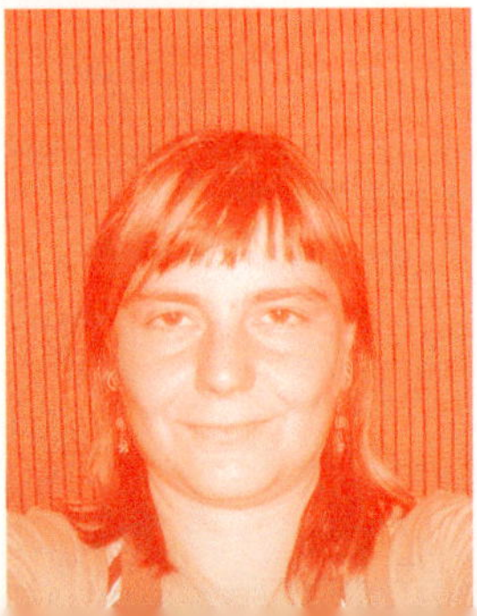
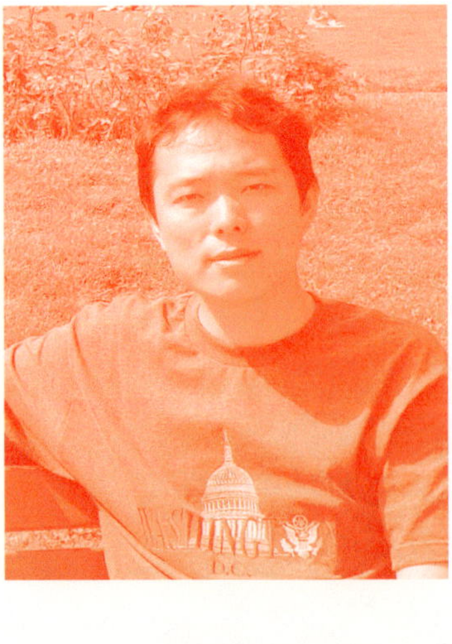

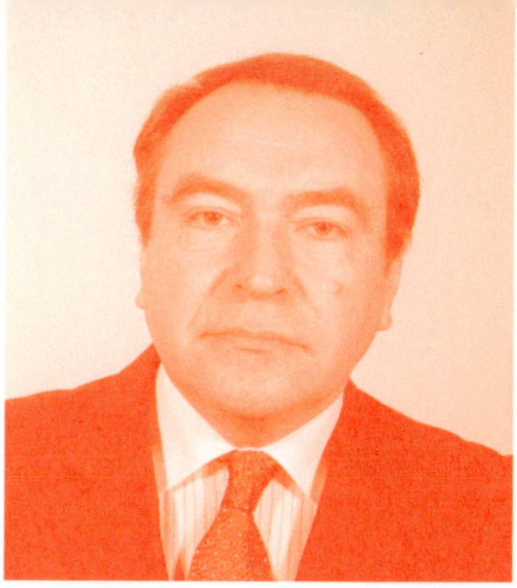
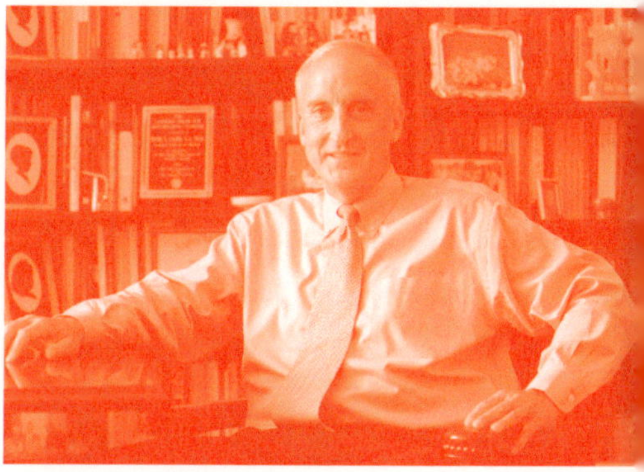
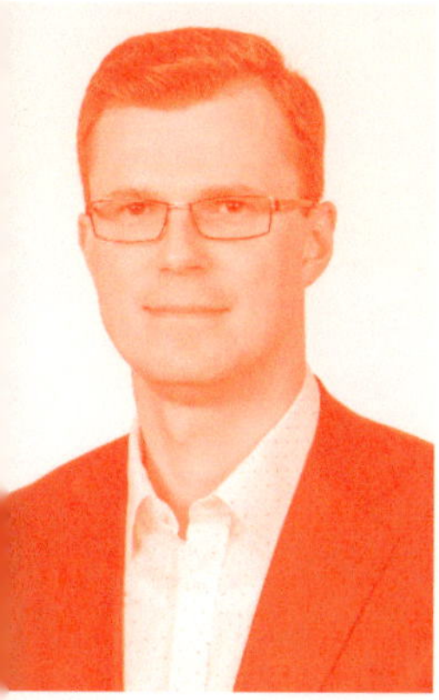
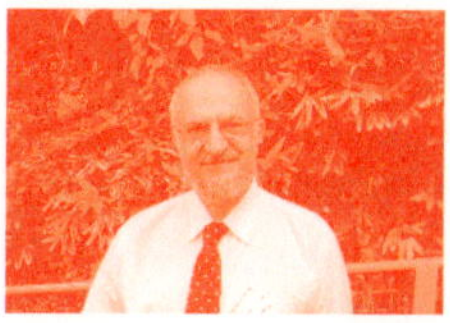
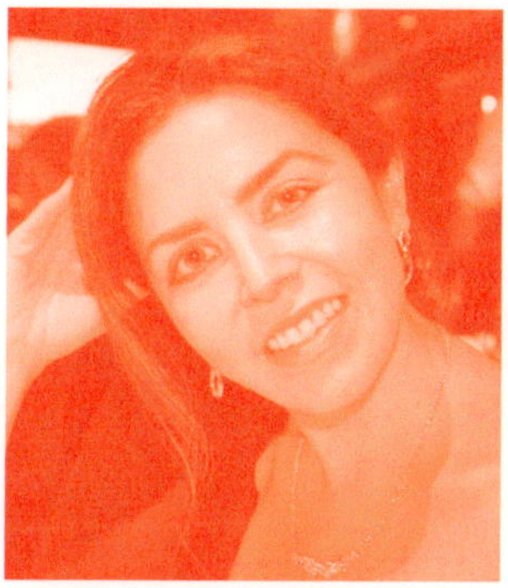

Supporting open minds since 2005

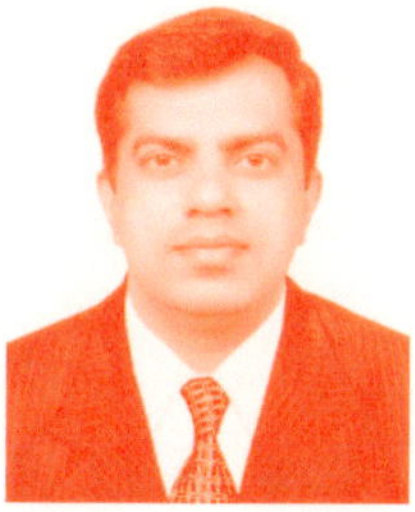
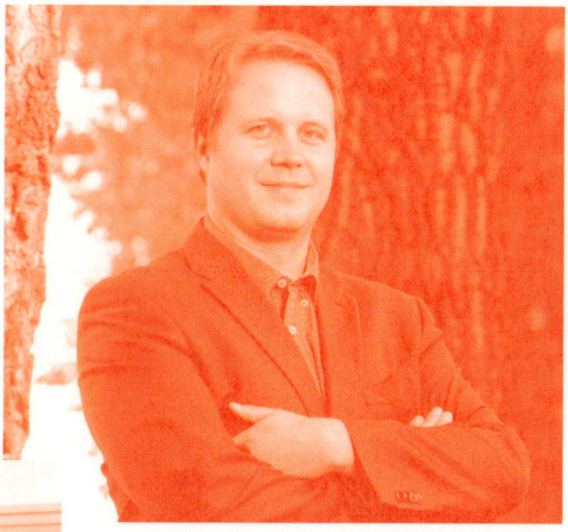
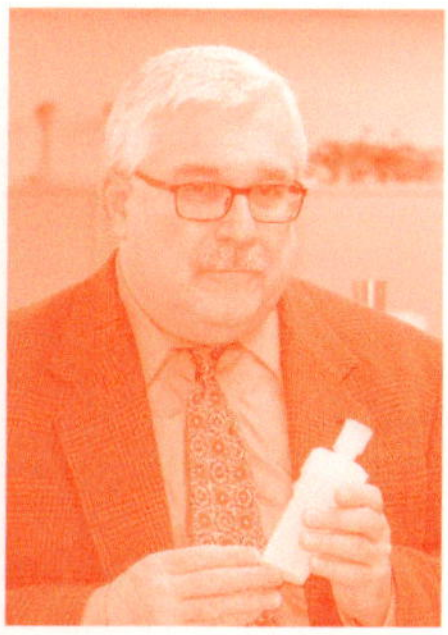
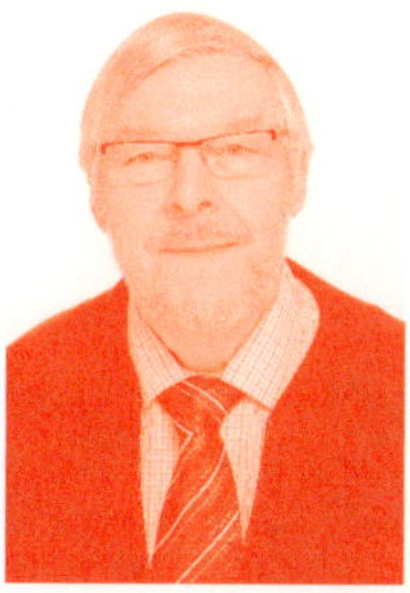
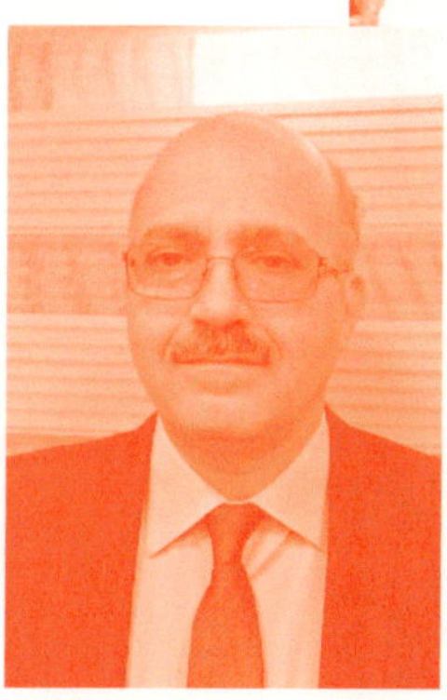
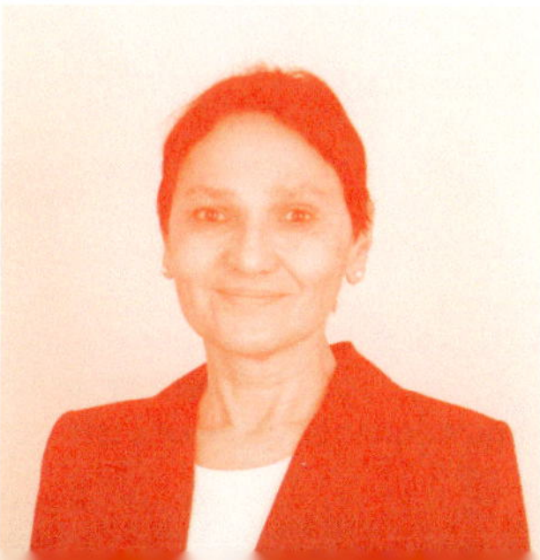
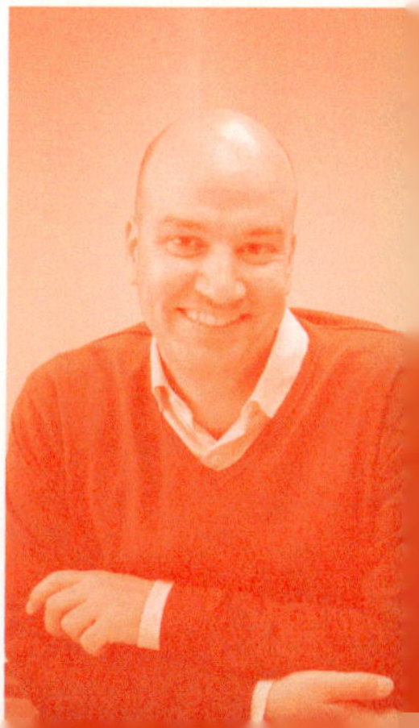

Chronobiology - The Science of Biological Time Structure
http://dx.doi.org/10.5772/intechopen.73428
Edited by Pavol Svorc

Contributors
Christian Focan, Marc Jarczok, Elisabeth Balint, Jennifer J McGrath, Harald Gündel, Okamoto-Uchida Yoshimi, Junko Izawa, Jun Hirayama, Akari Nishimura, Anastasiia Ledyaeva, Mikhail Ledyaev, Sergey Klauchek, Mohammad Rayees Dar, Abdul Roof Rather, Pavol Svorc

First published in London, United Kingdom, 2019 by IntechOpen
IntechOpen is the global imprint of INTECHOPEN LIMITED, registered in England and Wales, registration number: 11086078, 7th floor, 10 Lower Thames Street, London, EC3R 6AF, United Kingdom
Printed in Croatia

British Library Cataloguing-in-Publication Data
A catalogue record for this book is available from the British Library

Additional hard and PDF copies can be obtained from orders@intechopen.com

Chronobiology - The Science of Biological Time Structure
Edited by Pavol Svorc
p. cm.
Print ISBN 978-1-78984-900-4
Online ISBN 978-1-78984-901-1
eBook (PDF) ISBN 978-1-83962-277-9

Meet the editor

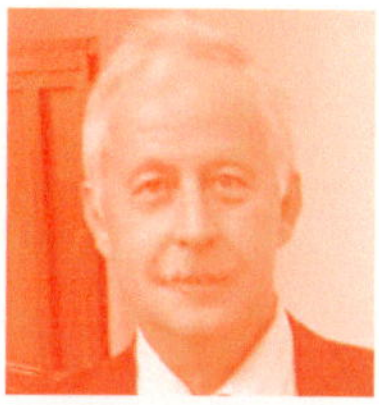

Pavol Svorc, Associate Professor of Normal and Patological Physiology, Doctor of the Natural Sciences, Philosophe Doctor, works at the Medical Faculty, Šafarik's University, in Košice. From 2011 until 2014 was Head of the Institute of Physiology and Pathophysiology, Medical Faculty, University of Ostrava, Czech Republic. He is a member of the committee for Human Physiology and Patophysiology in Jessenius Medical Faculty in Martin and of the committee for Neuroscience in the Medical Faculty in Ostrava. Currently, he is a visiting associate professor in the Medical Faculty in Ostrava, Ostrava University. His research focuses on chronobiology of the cardiovascular system, autonomic nervous system, and anesthesia. He has authored several international journal articles and book chapters, and participated in 129 conferences and workshops worldwide.

Contents

Preface

Chronobiology is the science investigating and objectively quantifying the mechanisms of the biological time structure, including the rhythmic manifestations of life. The disturbance of the temporal structure of the living organism leads to disturbed harmony between biological rhythms and the rhythm of the external environment often resulting in a cyclic course of various diseases.

A general view of the importance of chronobiology can be seen in the chapter „Time structure of the functional organization of living systems" by Mohammad Rayees Dar and Abdul Roof Rather. The authors describe the reality that there is a temporal biological system in living organisms that controls, synchronizes, and coordinates all body systems to external rhythmic changes. The authors present examples from everyday physiology and clinical medicine, where rhythmic phenomena can be encountered, as well as the meaning, perspectives, and representation of chronobiology in all scientific biological disciplines. More detailed issues of control of circadian rhythms are discussed in the chapter „Light-dependent regulation of circadian clocks in vertebrates" by Junko et al., where the authors analyze cellular-clock regulation in mammals and point out the specifics of cellular-clock regulation in zebrafish (direct synchronization of peripheral cellular clocks in addition to central cellular clocks by light).

In the cardiovascular system, practically all measurable functions exhibit circadian oscillations. The importance of dosing of antihypertensive drugs over time is receiving increased attention. The authors Narsingh Verma et al. in the chapter „Blood pressure variability and its clinical implications" discuss this problem in more detail and point to the fact that this type of therapy may be important because of the greater incidence of cardiovascular events in the early morning hours, in association with increases in blood pressure, heart rate, cardiac ischemia, enhanced platelet aggregability, and plasma catecholamines. Also important are the facts about dippers and nondippers and their relationship to other cardiovascular diseases whose predominance is in the early morning hours. The clinical physiology of children and older people refers to the differences that arise during ontogenesis in the endocrine system that in turn affects physiological functions. The authors Sheveleva et al. in the chapter "Circadian rhythm of blood pressure in children and adolescents" express the idea that formation of the circadian organization of the vegetative mechanisms that underlie the formation of daily arterial pressure profile probably depend on age.

Jarczok et al. in "Circadian rhythms of the autonomic nervous system—scientific implication and practical implementation" discuss the practical application of circadian heart rate variability (HRV) patterns, for example, at different risk states and diseases, including depression, where reduced HRV parameters and circadian rhythm disorders have been reported. The inflammatory reflex is a physiological mechanism through which the vagus nerve regulates immune function. In the chapter, there are a few examples confirming that 24-hour measurement of HRV may be a practical tool in prevention. This statement is supported by examples with intact chronobiology and then examples with clear disorders. Finally, it is emphasized that although HRV evaluation is not disease specific, it can be a tool for monitoring overall health, e.g. before and after treatment, and serve as a tool for demonstrating the patient's physiological responses to its specific environmental stimuli. Hence, HRV seems to be a suitable psychosomatic marker.

Focan et al. in the chapter „Integration of chronobiological concepts for NSCLC management?" point to the importance of biological rhythms regarding carcinogenesis and molecular biology in animal or human situations. Results support clearly the hypothesis that circadian rhythm disruption plays an important role in lung tumorogenesis, as well as a link between circadian epigenetic regulation and cancer development. These findings also suggest that circadian disruption induces the progression of malignant tumors via a WNT signaling pathway in models involving tumor cells similar to those encountered in human nonsmall cell lung carcinoma (NSCLC). Experimental and clinical data consider taking into account the temporal dimension („circadian") for the prevention and management of NSCLC. This type of observation illustrates that the circadian system is involved in the protection and restoration of tumor cells.

In the chapter „Impact of shift work on sleep problems, hormonal changes, and features of metabolic syndrome in industrial workers" Fadia Zyada addresses and describes the results of several authors who compared the levels of individual hormones in night shift workers and in morning and afternoon shift workers, in relation to sleep problems and features of metabolic syndrome, such as body mass index (BMI), type II diabetes, and cardiovascular problems. The overview of the results is interesting because it is concluded that night shift is the only independent predictor for hormone imbalance for shift workers rather than BMI, type II diabetes, cardiovascular problems, disturbed sleep, and sleep problems.

Circadian disruption may occur, and may be the result of a phase shifts in the oscillation of the circadian and activity-controlled physiological processes, or can be induced by factors related to periodic inputs: low contrast between day and night synchronizing signals; zeitgebers with different periods or unusual phasing; orzeitgeber shifts (jet lag syndrome, shift work). It can also be induced by factors related to oscillators: the uncoupling between the different oscillators inside the suprachiasmatic nucleus, the uncoupling between the central and peripheral oscillators, or clock gene functional alterations. This chronobiological pathology can be induced by factors related to outputs: for example, nocturnal melatonin suppression or loss of cortisol rhythmicity. Many pathological states can be promoted or impaired as a consequence of circadian disruption. This book includes chapters on recent research not only in the field of normal human chronobiology but also in experimental and clinical medicine.

Pavol Švorc
Department of Physiology,
Medical Faculty Safarik's University,
Kosice, Slovak Republic

Section 1

Introduction

Chapter 1

Introductory Chapter: Chronobiology - The Science of Biological Time Structure

Pavol Švorc

1. Introduction

Both humans and most animal species on our planet are exposed to regular alternations of light and darkness, with a constant periodicity of 24 h throughout their lifetime. This regular alternation of light and dark affects not only human biological systems but also the social organization of behavior. Processes occurring in the human organism, which are dependent on the periodic alteration and alternation of environmental factors, potentially affect the blind and those employed in shift work and "nocturnal types," whose habits deviate from the usual mode of most individuals. The mode of alternating light and darkness is different at the equator, behind the polar circles, and also at transitions across multiple time zones. The effect of such light modes is manifested in periodic changes in several physiological functions and biological rhythms exhibited at every level of life—in single cells, tissues, organs, and, ultimately, physiological systems of organisms.

Changes in the external environment, such as those of the weather or atmospheric conditions, can be **unpredictable**; therefore, organisms need systems that directly respond to changing environments. However, there are also **predictable** changes, which are the result of specific planetary movements such as the day-night cycle (rotation of the earth on its axis), the cycle of the moon (cycle of the moon around the earth), or annual cycles (cycle of the earth around the sun). For these predicable changes, organisms have specific mechanisms that generate endogenous biological rhythms corresponding directly to certain periodicities in the environment. They are not directly dependent on the rhythmicities of environment but only use the periodic information from the environment to synchronize biological oscillations with cycles of environment.

2. Biological rhythms and homeostasis

Biological rhythms are sequences of events that are repeated over time in the same manner and with the same interval; in other words, they are predictable in time. Biorhythms of organisms are the result of adaptation to changes in the environment, which is highly variable and exhibits variation in many factors. Chronobiology is the science investigating and objectively quantifying the mechanisms of biological time structure, including the rhythmic manifestations of life.

Because medicine is, in large part, based on homeostatic principles, the following scheme may be regarded as representative.

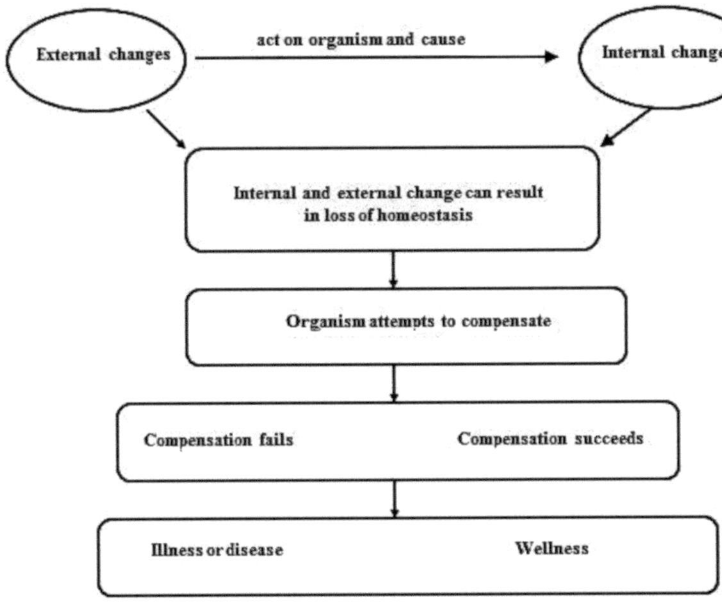

The survival of the animal in a highly periodic "day-night" environment, therefore, depends on the approximate timing of its reactions. Physiological systems must integrate and subsequently influence the responses of each system to different times of the day. Therefore, the traditional concept of homeostasis began to change. The **old concept of homeostasis** states that physiological variables are relatively constant only in a narrow physiological range throughout the day, which is essential for health. All organs and tissues of the body perform functions to maintain these constant conditions. However, the traditional concept of homeostasis involves no time dependence on the following:

- Results of diagnostic tests
- Occurrence or worsening of disease manifestations
- Pharmacokinetics of drugs
- Sensitivity to drugs
- Sensitivity to drugs in terms of pharmacodynamic—either therapeutic or side effect—drug properties

In contrast, the new concept of homeostasis states that physiological variables oscillate and are adjusted only to a narrow physiological range throughout the day, which is essential for health, and all organs and tissues of the body perform functions to maintain these constant conditions.

3. Distribution of biological rhythms

Exogenous rhythms: exogenous rhythms are oscillations of the passive system that depend on periodic stimulus from the external environment to which the organism synchronizes with these rhythmical changes. They are only observed within the circadian periodicity of the social or climatic environment.

Endogenous rhythms: endogenous rhythms are independently oscillating systems that are able to maintain their periodicity and also under constant nonperiodic conditions. Endogenous rhythms include:

Circadian rhythms: oscillate with a period of approximately 24 ± 4 h. They are one of the most frequently followed and studied rhythms. The term "circadian" was first used by professor [1] and has essentially two meanings. The first describes the day and night part of the day as a whole and the second as a cycle with a period of approximately 24 h.

Ultradian rhythms: oscillate with a period <20 h. The frequency of ultradian rhythms varies considerably from one species to another and from one parameter to another. In humans, several functions oscillate in 60–120 min intervals, and these rhythms are sometimes superimposed on other functions that oscillate at 3–5 min intervals.

Infradian rhythms: oscillate with the period >28 h. This term includes:

- *Circaseptan rhythms*: oscillate with a period of approximately 7 ± 3 days.
- *Circalunar rhythms*: rhythms with a period about 30 ± 5 days. Includes ovarial activity and the menstrual cycle in adult women.
- *Circannual rhythms*: oscillate with a period of approximately 1 year (±2 months), synchronized or desynchronized within a calendar year. It also includes *seasonal rhythms* that are the result of an adaptation process of living organisms to the environment. In certain species, reproductive functions are stimulated at specific moments in the annual cycle, thus optimizing the survival of the species. Although seasonal rhythms are also observed in humans, they do not exist to support species preservation.

4. Control of biological rhythms

The control of circadian rhythms occurs at the level of the retina (light input), the suprachiasmatic nuclei of the hypothalamus (clock genes), and the pineal gland (melatonin synthesis). Daylight or equivalent simulated light impacts retinal cells and passes the retinohypothalamic tract into the hypothalamic suprachiasmatic nuclei, which are referred to as the "internal clock." The current hypothesis regarding the multioscillatory structure of the circadian system [2] contains the following components [3]:

Inputs: environmental periodic cues can reset the phase of the central pacemaker so that the period and phase of circadian rhythms become coincident with the timing of external cues.

Central pacemakers: the suprachiasmatic nucleus or nuclei (SCN) is considered to be the major pacemaker of the circadian system, driving circadian rhythmicity in other brain areas and peripheral tissues by sending them neural and humoral signals.

Peripheral oscillators: most peripheral tissues and organs contain circadian oscillators. Usually they are under the control of the SCN; however, under some circumstances (e.g., restricted feeding, jet lag, and shift work), they can desynchronize from the SCN.

Outputs: central pacemakers and peripheral oscillators are responsible for the daily rhythmicity observed in most physiological and behavioral functions. Some of these over-rhythms (physical exercise, core temperature, sleep-wake cycle, and feeding time), in turn, provide feedback, which can modify the function of the SCN and peripheral oscillators.

5. Chronobiological terminology

The terminology accepted and approved in the field of chronobiology by The American Association of Medical Chronobiology and Chronotherapeutics describes aspects of biological rhythms that are often used in chronobiological texts, and for which no alternative terminology is suitable. This nomenclature was presented at the fourth Postgraduate Course of Medical Chronobiology and its Applications, held in Nevşehir [4]. As with other medical disciplines, the following terms must be introduced and should be accepted by specialists in this field. However, chronobiology is a rapidly evolving discipline, and, moreover, many of the established terms in the field of chronobiology remain unknown to many scientists and physicians who can benefit from applying chronobiological principles to their work.

Biological clocks: self-sustained oscillators that generate biological rhythms in the absence of external periodic input (e.g., at the gene level in cells).

Pacemaker: the functional unit capable of self-sustaining oscillations, which synchronize other rhythms or internal mechanisms, which sets the period and phase of the endogenous rhythm. They are oscillators (biological o'clock), which generate biological rhythms in the absence of external periodic inputs (e.g., at the gene level in individual cells). The hypothalamic suprachiasmatic nuclei are the dominant pacemaker of many circadian rhythms in mammals.

Synchronization: the state of a system when two or more variables exhibit periodicity with the same frequency, acrophase, and phasic relation. It refers to the adjustment of endogenous rhythm to external periodic influences. This influence is mediated by the synchronizer (**zeitgeber**)—the environmental periodicity determining the temporal placement of a biological rhythm along an appropriate time scale.

Human synchronizers can be:

- knowledge of the time of day
- light-dark cycle
- social contacts
- sleep-wake cycle
- time of eating
- electromagnetic field, gravitational field, and cosmic radiation

Desynchronization (internal): a state in which two or more previously synchronized variables within the same organism (endogenous rhythms) cease to exhibit different time relations.

Desynchronization (external): desynchronization of biological (endogenous) rhythm from an environmental cycle.

Free-running rhythms: endogenous rhythms with their own periods, which also persist under conditions in which the periodicity of the external environment is modified or eliminated.

Phase shifts: if the period or timing of a dominant synchronizer changes, endogenous circadian rhythms, but synchronized with environment, follow a shift of their synchronizer and display phase advances or phase delays. The rhythms adapt to this new condition in a time—re-entrainment.

Phase advance and phase delay: involves the earlier or later occurrence of a rhythm's phase, usually acrophase.

Entrainment: coupling of two rhythms of the same frequency to one of them (the entraining agent or synchronizer) determining the phase of the other. It is coupling of endogenous rhythms to an environmental oscillator of the same frequency or determination of the phase of biological rhythms by an internal pacemaker.

Self-sustained oscillation: a system that can make use of a constant source of energy and is able to continue to oscillate without outside energy input.

Episodic variation: apparently irregular (nonrhythmic) variation of a biological variable (e.g., episodic secretion of certain hormones).

Reference rhythm and marker rhythm: is the rhythm of one variable used as a time reference for other rhythms.

6. Clinical medicine: chronomedicine

After the discovery of the mechanism of circadian rhythm, functioning did not last long, and numerous studies were carried out describing their impact on the etiopathogenesis of diseases as well as the possibility of their application in therapy. Even in the 3–6 weeks after birth, the internal clocks are gradually synchronized with 24-h period. In the greatest extent, the influence of lighting shares on this synchronization, but the role of melatonin, which is found in breast milk only at night, is also discussed. However, circadian rhythms also occur in the blind people, and even 50–75% blind people indicate that they suffer by sleep disorders.

Periodic phenomena are encountered in many studies investigating various diseases. Very often, many symptoms or significant remissions exhibit a cyclic course. The time structure of living organisms is the source of these phenomena: accurate intermodulation over time, changing biological variables, and similar. If the harmony between and among biological rhythms is disrupted or disordered, the subjects themselves detect susceptibility to the disease or the disease itself. It is necessary to capture these different situations by monitoring the biological phenomenon during the day and to estimate the periodicity of the system using precise statistical methods.

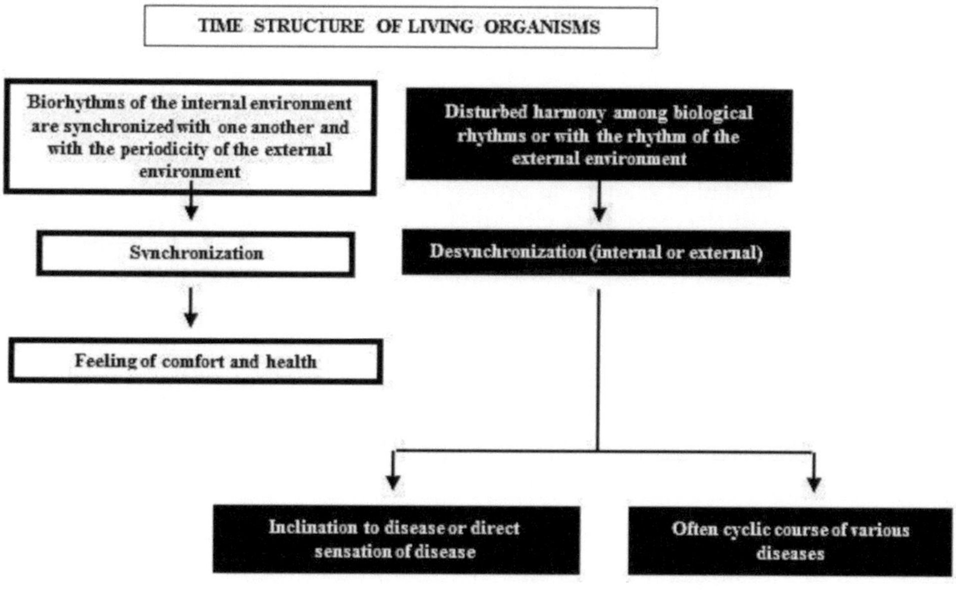

The question, then, is when to perform laboratory examinations or diagnostic tests. For example, plasma cortisol exhibits a circadian rhythm. Although secretion increases in response to the stressful stimulus, it is spontaneously released during the day with peak values around 4:00–6:00 in the morning, with a gradual decrease during the day to the lowest values that fall between 23:00 and 2:00 a.m. If the value of "normal" occurs at approximately 08:00 h, approximately 20:00 h would represent Cushing syndrome. If the value of "normal" occurs at approximately 20:00, 08:00 h would represent Addison disease. From a circadian perspective, the conclusion is adrenal cortex hyperactivity would be diagnosed only if a high plasma cortisol concentration was found in the evening and adrenal cortex insufficiency if low levels were found in the morning.

What can be a recommendation? Creation of "individual chronobiological profile" to use of improvement of the diagnostic test accuracy problems at which is not possible to suppose that internal circadian time is equal to the real time:

- At the transitions through more time zones (jetlag syndrome)
- In shift workers
- In students during examination periods
- During hospitalization—at the relative constant levels of murmurs, light, and at the continual work of nurse
- Resulting in the disorders of the circadian orientation, although the normal phase orientation is at the start

7. Circadian disruption: disruption of biological timing

The circadian system optimizes daytime behavior and physiology and is organized hierarchically with central clocks in the SCN that are primarily synchronized by light. Currently, we are commonly exposed to less light and more night-light due to artificial lighting, which can negatively impact the organization of the circadian system and disturb sleep, resulting in extensive adverse effects on metabolic health. Interrupted sleep, for example, supports the increase of energy intake and reduction of energy expenditure, which may affect healthy eating. Experiments have also demonstrated that circadian deviations can lead to several metabolic abnormalities [5].

Circadian rhythm disturbance may occur from the level of the molecular clock (which regulates cellular activity) to the mismatch between behavioral and environmental cycles [5]. It is the result of a phase shift in the oscillation of the circadian and activity-controlled physiological processes. A recent study found that chronic disruption of one of the most basic circadian (daily) rhythms—the day-night cycle—leads to weight gain, impulsivity, slower thinking, and other physiological and behavioral changes in mice, similar to those observed in individuals who engage in shift work or experience jet lag.

This circadian pathology can be induced by factors related to **inputs** such as low contrast between day and night synchronizing signals (continuous light, frequent snacking, low levels of physical exercise), by zeitgebers with different periods or unusual phasing (i.e., light at night, nocturnal eating, nocturnal physical activity), or by zeitgeber shifts (i.e., daylight saving time, crossing time zones, shift work).

Shift work: because individuals in various occupations often work at night, they are exposed to an extraordinary risk for circadian rhythm and sleep disturbances [6–9].

Shift workers are also susceptible to other health disorders such as gastrointestinal problems [10], and exposure to work-related changes can be associated with the risk for certain diseases, including breast cancer and metabolic syndrome [11, 12].

Jetlag: in addition to shift work, jetlag also induces circadian rhythm and sleep disturbances. Although the health consequences of frequent jetlag are ambiguous [13], any harmful effects of jetlag-induced circadian rhythm and sleep disturbances are becoming more widespread as an increasing number of passengers are projected to cross multiple time zones. While shift work and jetlag bring a clear disruption of the circadian system and sleep, even "normal" work hours can result in a smoother imbalance of circadian rhythm and sleep deprivation, especially among evening chronotypes. This is because many individuals use alarms to produce wakefulness when sleep would otherwise occur [5].

Other sources of circadian disruption can be unusual photoperiod (polar regions), circadian rhythm sleep (wake disorders [non-24-h sleep-wake disorders], senescence, disease states [Alzheimer's disease, Smith-Magenis syndrome, Parkinson disease]), and pregnancy, menopause, mental health problems, or medications.

Circadian pathology can be induced by factors related to oscillators such as the uncoupling between the different oscillators inside the SCN caused by aging and the uncoupling between the central and peripheral oscillators or clock gene functional alterations result in circadian disruption or can be induced by factors related to outputs such as nocturnal melatonin suppression and loss of cortisol rhythmicity, which are also chronodisrupters. Many pathological states can be induced or impaired as consequence of circadian disruption [3].

Common circadian rhythm disorders include:

Jetlag or rapid time zone change syndrome: individuals with this syndrome exhibit symptoms that include excessive sleepiness and a lack of daytime alertness in those who travel across time zones.

Shift work sleep disorder: this sleep disorder affects individuals who frequently rotate shifts or work at night.

Delayed sleep phase syndrome (DSPS): this is a disorder of sleep timing. Individuals with DSPS tend to fall asleep very late at night and have difficulty waking up in time for work, school, or social engagements.

Advanced sleep phase disorder (ASPD): this is a disorder in which an individual goes to sleep earlier and wakes earlier than desired. ASPD results in symptoms of evening sleepiness, going to bed earlier (e.g., between 6:00 and 9:00 p.m.) and waking up earlier than desired (e.g., between 1:00 and 5:00 a.m.).

Non-24-h sleep-wake disorder: this disorder frequently affects those that are totally blind because the circadian clock is set by the light-dark cycle over a 24-h period. In non-24-h sleep-wake disorder, the cycle is disturbed. The disorder results in drastically reduced sleep time and quality at night and problems with sleepiness during daylight hours.

Some behavioral and pharmaceutical interventions balance the adverse effects of circadian rhythm and sleep disorders; however, some of the beneficial effects of these interventions may be independent of the circadian system and sleep. Because understanding of the relationships between the healthy phases of the SCN and peripheral clock systems is poorly characterized, clarifying these relationships may help to personalize chronobiotic prescriptions, some of which still require safety and efficacy studies. It is then necessary to compare these interventions and to assess which are most effective and under what circumstances [5].

Currently, it is no longer sufficient to classify health as the potential ability of an organism to cope with the varying effects of the environment without disturbing biologically important functions. We have the resources and a relatively accurate statistical methodology that enables us to assess the maximum and minimum functional capacities of each functional system at any time.

Author details

Pavol Švorc
Department of Physiology, Medical Faculty Safarik's University, Košice, Slovak Republic

*Address all correspondence to: svorc@upjs.sk

References

[1] Halberg F. Circadian system phase—An aspect of temporal morphology, producers and illustrative examples. In: von Mayerbach H, editor. The Cellular Aspects of Biorhythms. Berlin: Springer; 1967. pp. 20-48

[2] Vaze KM, Nikhil KL, Sharma VK. Circadian rhythms. Resonance. 2014;**19**:175-189

[3] Garaulet M, Ordovás JM, Madrid JA. The chronobiology, etiology and pathophysiology of obesity. International Journal of Obesity. 2010;**34**:1667-1683

[4] Course Booklet from 4th Postgraduate the Course of Medical Chronobiology and its Applications in Nevsehir, Turkey; 2006

[5] Potter GDM, Skene DJ, Arendt J, Cade JE, Grant PJ, Hardie LJ. Circadian rhythm and sleep disruption: Causes, metabolic consequences, and countermeasures. Endocrine Reviews. 2016;**37**:584-608

[6] Folkard S. Do permanent night workers show circadian adjustment? A review based on the endogenous melatonin rhythm. Chronobiology International. 2008;**25**:215-224

[7] Arendt J, Middleton B, Williams P, Francis G, Luke C. Sleep and circadian phase in a ship's crew. Journal of Biological Rhythms. 2006;**21**:214-221

[8] Arendt J. Shift work: Coping with the biological clock. Occupational Medicine (London). 2010;**60**:10-20

[9] Axelsson J, Akerstedt T, Kecklund G, Lowden A. Tolerance to shift work—How does it relate to sleep and wakefulness? International Archives of Occupational and Environmental Health. 2004;**77**:121-129

[10] Knutsson A, Bøggild H. Gastrointestinal disorders among shift workers. Scandinavian Journal of Work, Environment & Health. 2010;**36**:85-95

[11] Wang F, Yeung KL, Chan WC, Kwok CC, Leung SL, Wu C, et al. A meta-analysis on dose-response relationship between night shift work and the risk of breast cancer. Annals of Oncology. 2013;**24**:2724-2732

[12] Wang F, Zhang L, Zhang Y, Zhang B, He Y, Xie S, et al. Meta-analysis on night shift work and risk of metabolic syndrome. Obesity Reviews. 2014;**15**:709-720

[13] Hammer GP, Auvinen A, De Stavola BL, Grajewski B, Gundestrup M, Haldorsen T, et al. Mortality from cancer and other causes in commercial airline crews: A joint analysis of cohorts from 10 countries. Occupational and Environmental Medicine. 2014;**71**:313-322

Section 2

Time Structure of the Functional Organization of Living System

Chapter 2

Chronobiology and Its General Perspectives

Mohammad Rayees Dar and Abdul Roof Rather

Abstract

As a significance of the earth's rotation about its axis approximately every 24 hours, most organisms on this planet are subjected to probable variations of light and temperature. A diverse range of species, from cyanobacteria to humans, evolved internal biological clocks that allow for the anticipation of these daily variations. The field of chronobiology, the study of the rhythms in plants and animals, was limited to botanists for centuries. Only recently during the last decades, the research was expanded to include animals and later even human beings. Rhythms have been recognized and associated to the fluctuation of day and night and to the succession of the seasons. Nowadays, chronobiology has developed into a multidisciplinary field in which scientists are involved in basic research as well as in applied topics.

Keywords: chronobiology, circadian rhythm, infradian, ultradian, chronophysiology

1. Introduction

Most organisms on this planet are subject to the significance of earth's rotation around its axis, approximately every 24 hours, for probable variations of light and temperature. A vast range of species, from cyanobacteria to human beings, evolved internal biological clocks that permit for the eagerness of these daily variations. Thus, physiology and functions of an organism are primarily intertwined with this geophysical cycle. An astronomer in 1729, whose name was Jean-Jacques d'Ortousde Mairan presented early impending into this evolutionary relationship between inner physiology and the geophysical cycle, he reported that daily leaf activities in heliotrope plants persist in constant darkness [1]. In 1959, another scientist whose name was Franz Halberg give emphasis to the endogenous nature of biological clocks and coined the term circadian, that refer to daily rhythms which are truly endogenously generated, i.e., rhythms having a time period of about 24 hours that continue to vary in the absence of any environmental input [2]. The term circadian comes from the Latin *circa*, meaning "around" and *dies*, "day," meaning "approximately a day." It is regulated by circadian clocks. A recognized intrinsic property of single cells has been named as rhythm making, which was determined by an intracellular molecular oscillator based on transcriptional/post translational negative response loops. Endogenous variations are synchronized to the environment under common conditions, and is usually considered that biological clock present an adaptive advantage by guarantying that internal biochemical and physiological progression of an organism's in accumulation to actions, are optimally tailored to the neighboring atmosphere [3, 4].

The study of rhythms in animals and plants was restricted to botanists for centuries but in modern times, the search could be extended to incorporate animals and later on even human beings. Rhythms have been recognized and attached to the variability of day and night and to the progression of the seasons. Currently, this study has been developed into a multidimensional field in which scientists are concerned with fundamental examination as well as in practical areas. Chronobiology, as a field of biology study, the very cyclic phenomena in living beings and their modifications that are linked to solar- and lunar-related rhythms. Such cycles are known as biological rhythms [5]. Chronobiology has it origin from Greek, comprise of two words *chromos*, meaning "time" and *biology*, which means "study of life." Terms like *chronomics* and *chronome* which are related to it have been used in some cases to explain either the pertinent molecular mechanisms involved in the phenomena of chronobiology or to explore the most assessable aspects of chronobiology, and in particular where the assessment of cycles between the living beings is required. Everyday physiology is described by chronobiology under ordinary conditions and also after the standardization or constancy. This may be, as far as possible, comprised of environmental temperature, lighting, the availability of food and other manipulable local conditions [6]. Chronobiology is an important tool of new biology rather of a new and cohesive science. Indeed, rhythmic studies in and around us provide basis for a broader transdisciplinary science which includes all branches of medicine, chemistry, biology, physics, sociology, and in particular cosmology.

Chronobiological studies include comparative anatomy, physiology, genetics, molecular biology and behavior of organisms within biological rhythms mechanics but are not limited to these areas. Other aspects include epigenetics, development, reproduction, ecology and evolution. Chronobiology is an interdisciplinary field of study and research, which interacts with medical and other research fields such as sleep medicine, endocrinology, geriatrics (branch of medicine that focuses on health promotion, prevention and treatment of disease and disability in life), sports medicine, space medicine and photoperiodism [7–9]. The factual biology of chronobiology rests in the wide variety of procedures that are controlled by the circadian clock. Even though this biology plays an essential role at the level of the whole organism, it derives, finally, from clock-driven fluctuations in physiology, and quite often in gene expression, that come about at the level of individual cells. For many essential biological processes the differences of the timing and space in natural activity in living beings takes place, for example, in animals (cellular regeneration, eating, hibernating, sleeping, mating, migration, etc.), in plants (photosynthetic reactions, leaf movements, etc.), and in microbial organisms such as fungi and protozoa. These essential processes have even been found in bacteria, mainly in the blue-green algae. Circadian rhythm is the most dynamic rhythm in the field of chronobiology, an approximately 24-hours cycle revealed by biological processes in all the above mentioned organisms [10].

Based on routine cycles during the 24-hour day, the circadian rhythms can further be classified as: (a) diurnal, daytime activity of an organism, (b) nocturnal, nighttime activity of the organisms, and (c) crepuscular, organisms which are active at the dawn and dusk hours. The control process of circadian rhythms is defined as endogenous, and other biological cycles may be controlled by exogenous signals. While multi-tropic systems may flair rhythms driven by the circadian clock of one of the members (which may also be predisposed or reorganized by external factors) [11].

Other important cycles studied, include (a) infradian rhythms are longer than a day, for example, the reproduction or annual cycles of migration in many plants and animals or menstrual cycles in humans, (b) ultradian rhythms are shorter than

24-hours, for example, 3-hour growth hormone production cycle, 4-hour nasal cycle and/or 90-minute REM cycle, (c) tidal rhythms are roughly 12.4-hour transition from high to low and vice versa and are usually seen in marine life, (d) lunar rhythms follow the lunar month (29.5 days) and is related to the modulations of the level of tides across the lunar cycle [12], and (e) gene fluctuations have different activity cycles for acrophase (the period during which the process is more active) and bathyphase (when the process is less active). How high or low the process gets is measured by the amplitude. Some genes are more expressed during certain hours than other hours, e.g., cortisol, melatonin, etc. [13].

2. Chronobiology subdivisions

Some subdivisions of chronobiology are:

1. Chronophysiology: the fiction of "baselines" in an imaginary homeostasis is replaced by chronophysiology through dynamic parameters and competent feedbacks and feed forwards in organisms by feed sideward in a collateral hierarchy of living things and of external-internal interactions. As far as, time analysis is concerned the same stimulus has different effects at various predictable stages of a rhythm's timescale [14]. Responses in the form of data can then be quantified by using reference values, for example, parametric and nonparametric sum of blood pressure and heart rate variability over time, of people of different gender, age and ethnicity in health [3, 4].

2. Chronohygiene: it is meant through pre-habilitation, which means it detects elevation of risk by analysing a variation of rhythm characteristics before and after deviations in the average. Thus, before pathology becomes overt and symptomatic by a conventional approach relying on a normal range, it recognizes an increase in the risk of disease and covert pathology, e.g., by monitoring the circulation parameters of body such as blood pressure and heart rate of an individual in time, combining it with chronobiological data examination, it detects certain unfavorable collections of sequential variables early before hypertension occurs. Pre-habilitation deals with the enhancement of health by means of prophylactic interference with a purpose of decreasing the risk of diseases, it relies on the procedures like as the scheduling of food intake [6]. Exercise, on the other hand, must not be scheduled to induce involuntary circadian blood pressure over swing. Likewise, prayer, meditation, self-hypnosis and other procedures employed could explore any kind of influence by the time structures of the organism and its environment. Meanwhile, socio environmental-organism interactions like those in close association with the about 10-years solar activity cycle (SAC) and/or extreme magnetic storms have effects that may ultimately lead to a space weather report and to corresponding preventive research. Gene studies and genome research which has found connections between genes and diseases may be complemented by the genome mapping with various characteristics such as the circadian periods, amplitudes and phases both in the more readily assessed 24-hour synchronized state and under the conditions of desynchronization or multiple synchronization [3, 4].

3. Chronotherapy: it refers to timing treatment in order to maximize the effects at the same time minimizing the undesired effects. Seeking possibilities, the treatment is timed to marker rhythms for each of the desired effect and for each of the undesired effect. Chronotherapy utilizes a set of different

parameters for cases like cancer, including physical markers, ranging from a chemical tumor marker or a tumor temperature and/or the bone marrow's integrity hematological gauges, and to gauge cardiotoxicity, vascular parameters among others. The chronobiologically interpreted ambulatory blood pressure monitoring may provide information regarding the need for treatment of vascular variability disorder along with its timing. This information could be about the confirmation of the desired as well as undesired effects and this may avoid the status quo with misdiagnosed vascular variability disorder [3, 4].

4. Medical chronobiology: being an emerging field of medicine, its prime concern is with two important issues (a) chronopathology deals with the effect of circadian rhythms and the indices of disease; and (b) chronopharmacology deals with the study of the circadian variability of efficacy and toxicity of various treatments for a wide variety of medical conditions [15].

In chronopathology additional biological systems and disease conditions are reflected on, it has turn out to be evident that many conditions, not all, have an expected circadian variation in activity or severity. For example, blood pressure is lowest at 3:00 am; epidermal mitosis is maximal at midnight. The same seizes to be true for disease states: asthma is bad at early morning, and cerebral hemorrhage hit the highest point in the evening. Asthma at night is likely one of the most studied medical disorders in which there are perfect chronobiological stages. More is the climax of incidence of biological variables and disease conditions, more efficient treatment techniques can be developed.

In the field of chronopharmacology, not only pharmacological agents handle natural rhythms, but the sufficient range of medicines along with their timing of administration and other therapies such as irradiation may have reflective effects upon their value and toxicity. By the management of drug at the suitable time of the day, the therapeutic benefits may be maximized and the toxic side effects may be minimized. Circadian rhythms have been verified in rate of metabolism and inactivation, along with differences in blood volume and extracellular fluid volume, ensuing in variable degrees of attenuation of the drug, susceptibility of the target organs to the circulating drug.

All included with the consequence of circadian difference in reply to a precise prescriptions and treatments. There is credible indication of the suggestion of taking into consideration time of the circadian rhythm in management of drug from clinical areas such as use of anesthetics and antiepileptic drugs, cancer chemotherapy, and steroid administration. Some specific examples of circadian variation are: (a) evening medication with diltiazem is more effective than other dosage schedules, and (b) constant intravenous infusion of heparin has a maximum anticoagulant effect between 4:00 and 8:00 am, with a minimum effect at noon, indicating that the laboratory control studies should be performed at fixed times. Very small work has been carried out on the circadian considerations of drugs operated in the treatment of sleep disorders till now as narcolepsy is an exceptional example of a sleep disorder. At present data is not available to help in planning the timing of medicine to maximize therapeutic outcomes and minimize toxicity of the drug. This concept presents a demanding novel prospect for research of drug therapy in sleep disorders.

Chronomolecular biology is itself a very vast area of study, which actively discuss the mechanisms, approaches and beyond as biological clocks. Pertinent to it, chronobiology in its broader aspect are the findings that infradians—such as half-weekly, weekly, circaparasemiannual, half-yearly, para-annual, transyearly, yearly and even transtridecadal modulations of the circadian rhythm characteristics—are now represented as having significant relations in disease and health. Infradians and some ultradians may be tied to the circadian system, as may be the development of a roundworm in the laboratory. In recent decades, chronobiology has exposed the truth of a temporal regulation system that synchronizes all body systems to environmental cycles, such as the day-night cycle. Hence, it is at present known that living organisms react proactively to environmental rhythmicity and for that reason prepare actively.

Author details

Mohammad Rayees Dar[1*] and Abdul Roof Rather[2]

1 Animal Physiology Division, National Dairy Research Institute, Karnal, Haryana, India

2 Department of Physical Education, Central University of Kashmir, Ganderbal, Jammu and Kashmir, India

*Address all correspondence to: rayeesr21@gmail.com

References

[1] Kreitzman L, Foster RG. Rhythms of Life: The Biological Clocks that Control the Daily Lives of every Living Thing. New Haven, Connecticut: Yale University Press; 2004. ISBN 0-300-10969-5

[2] Chandrashekaran MK. Biological rhythms research: A personal account. Journal of Biosciences. 1998;**23**:545

[3] Halberg F. Chronobiology: Methodological problems. Acta Medica Romana. 1980;**18**:399-440

[4] Halberg F. Quo vadis basic and clinical chronobiology: Promise for health maintenance. The American Journal of Anatomy. 1983;**168**:543-594

[5] DeCoursey PJ, Dunlap JC, Loros JJ. Chronobiology. Sunderland, Massachusetts, USA: Sinauer Associates Inc.; 2003. ISBN 978-0-87893-149-1

[6] Fuller PM, Lu J, Saper CB. Differential rescue of light- and food-entrainable circadian rhythms. Science. 2008;**320**(5879):1074-1077. DOI: 10.1126/science.1153277. PMC 3489954. PMID 18497298. Bibcode: 2008Sci.320.1074F [Accessed: 30 May 2008]

[7] Rossi EL, Lloyd D. Ultradian Rhythms in Life Processes: An Inquiry into Fundamental Principles of Chronobiology and Psychobiology. Springer, Berlin, Heidelberg: Springer-Verlag Berlin and Heidelberg GmbH & Co. K; 1992. ISBN 978-3-540-19746-1

[8] Hayes DK. Chronobiology: Its Role in Clinical Medicine, General Biology, and Agriculture. Hoboken, New Jersey, US: John Wiley & Sons; 1990. ISBN 978-0-471-56802-5

[9] Postolache TT. Sports Chronobiology, an Issue of Clinics in Sports Medicine. Philadelphia, US: Saunders; 2005. ISBN 978-1-4160-2769-0

[10] Dzogang F, Lightman S, Cristianini N. Diurnal variation of psychometric indicators in twitter content. PLoS One. 2018;**13**(6). DOI: 10.1371/journal.pone.0197002. eCollection

[11] Nelson RJ. An Introduction to Behavioral Endocrinology. Massachusetts: Sinauer Associates, Inc.; 2005. p. 587

[12] Frank DW, Evans JA, Gorman MR. Time-dependent effects of dim light at night on re-entrainment and masking of hamster activity rhythms. Journal of Biological Rhythms. 2010;**25**(2):103-112. DOI: 10.1177/0748730409360890

[13] Refinetti R. Circadian Physiology. 2nd ed. Boca Raton, FL: CRC Press, Taylor & Francis Group; 2006. p. 700. ISBN 0-8493-2233-2

[14] Refinetti R, Cornélissen G, Halberg F. Procedures for numerical analysis of circadian rhythms. Biological Rhythm Research. 2007;**38**(4):275-325. DOI: 10.1080/09291010 600903692

[15] Cornelissen G, Halberg F. Introduction to chronobiology. In: Medtronic Chronobiology Seminar #7; April 1994. Library of Congress Catalog Card #94-060580; 1994. p. 52. Available from: http://www.msi.umn.edu/~halberg/

Chapter 3

Light-Dependent Regulation of Circadian Clocks in Vertebrates

Izawa Junko, Yoshimi Okamoto-Uchida, Akari Nishimura and Jun Hirayama

Abstract

Circadian clocks are intrinsic time-tracking systems that endow organisms with a survival advantage. The core of the circadian clock mechanism is a cell-autonomous and self-sustained oscillator called a cellular clock, which operates via a transcription-/translation-based negative feedback loop. Under natural conditions, circadian clocks are entrained to a 24-hour day by environmental time cues, most commonly light. In mammals, circadian clocks are regulated by cellular clocks located in the central nervous system, such as the suprachiasmatic nucleus (SCN), and in other peripheral tissues. Importantly, mammals have no photoreceptors in the peripheral tissues; therefore the effect of light on peripheral clocks is indirect. By striking contrast, zebrafish peripheral cellular clocks are directly light responsive. This characteristic of the zebrafish cellular clock has contributed to the identification of molecules and signaling pathways that are involved in the light-dependent regulation of the cellular clock. Here, selected light-dependent regulatory mechanisms of circadian clocks in mammals and zebrafish are described.

Keywords: circadian clock, cellular clock, zebrafish, light, photolyase

1. Introduction

Circadian clocks constitute ubiquitous processes that regulate various biochemical and physiological events that occur with 24-hour periodicity, even in the absence of external cues [1]. The exact timing of this rhythm is established by cell-autonomous mechanisms, called cellular clocks, which are controlled by a transcription-/translation-based negative feedback loop [2, 3]. In both vertebrates and invertebrates, cellular clocks are scattered throughout their bodies; thus, the circadian system comprises both central and peripheral oscillators [4].

To guarantee that an organism's behavior remains tied to the rhythms of its environment, the circadian clock must respond to environmental stimuli to be reset [5]. The main cue for animals is light, which is provided by the day-night cycle. It has been proposed that in mammals the light-induced resetting of the circadian clock is dependent on transcription activation in the suprachiasmatic nucleus (SCN), where the central clock is located [6]. The mammalian route for the regulation of the circadian clock by light uses the retinohypothalamic tract (RHT), which connects directly to the central clock located in the SCN [7]. This makes it difficult to understand the mechanisms underlying light regulation of the circadian clock at a cellular level. Thus, although changes in gene expression have been implicated in the light-induced phase shift of the circadian clock [6, 8], the induction of the expression of clock genes by light and the exact mechanism by which these gene products work remain to be elucidated at the cellular level.

Zebrafish peripheral clocks display a striking characteristic in that they are directly light responsive [9, 10]. Light induces the expression of clock genes and the circadian expression of several clock-related genes in zebrafish peripheral cells [11]. In addition, zebrafish embryonic cell lines can recapitulate the light-response characteristics of a vertebrate clock. In these cell lines, the oscillations of clock gene expression can be entrained to a new light-dark cycle, showing that cultured zebrafish cells have the clock components required for light-induced circadian clock resetting, and the cultured cell system thus provides a valuable tool for studying the light-dependent regulation of the circadian clock at a cellular level [12, 13]. Zebrafish cellular clocks can be studied in cultured cells, which facilitate the study of the photic responses of clock genes encoding cellular-clock regulators, and have revealed cellular signaling pathways that are involved in the light-dependent regulation of the cellular clock [14–18]. Additionally, an increased understanding of light-dependent cellular-clock regulation in zebrafish has suggested intriguing associations among the circadian clock, DNA repair, and cell cycle control [19–23].

Here we describe selected light-dependent regulatory aspects of vertebrate circadian machinery.

2. Cellular-clock regulation in mammals

In mammals, the cellular clock comprises the CLOCK, NPAS2, BMAL1, BMAL2, PER1, PER2, CRY1, and CRY2 proteins [1, 24]. These cellular clock components are called clock proteins. CLOCK or NPAS2 proteins heterodimerize with BMALs to form an active transcription complex that transactivates clock-controlled genes, including *Crys* and *Pers*. Once the CRY and PER proteins have been translated, they are translocated to the nucleus, where they inhibit CLOCK (NPAS2):BMAL-mediated transcription through a direct protein-protein interaction, setting up the rhythmic gene expression that drives the circadian clock. The CLOCK(NPAS2):BMAL complex also stimulates expression of the clock-controlled genes (Ccgs) to regulate various elements of physiology. This accounts in part for the presence of circadian rhythms in a variety of physiological processes [25]. Although the relatively straightforward mechanism of positive and negative feedback loops is necessary to establish and maintain circadian clocks, cellular clocks have further levels of complexity, including posttranscriptional regulation, posttranslational modification, chromatin remodeling, availability and stability of clock proteins, and regulation of intracellular localization. These regulatory mechanisms provide an interface that can be used as an entry point for stimuli that can reset or control the clock. In addition, genetic studies of genes encoding cellular-clock regulators have revealed distinct roles for clock proteins in regulating circadian clocks, as well as direct links between the circadian clock and various pathologies [26–28].

3. Photoreceptors for circadian-clock regulation in mammals

Circadian clocks regulate various biochemical, physiological, and behavioral processes with a periodicity of approximately 24 hours. Under natural conditions, circadian rhythms are entrained to this 24-hour day by environmental time cues, with light level being the most important [5]. The eye is the principal mediator of light input to the central clock in mammals. Rods and cones receive visual information within the retina [29, 30] (**Figure 1**). These cells, however, are dispensable for photoreception of circadian clocks. Indeed, rodents that lack classical visual responses are still capable of circadian photoentrainment [31]. Retrograde tracing experiments have identified retinal cells projecting to the SCN through the RHT, but not to the visual centers of the brain [32]. These cells constitute a small subset of retinal ganglion cells (RGCs) localized in the ganglion cell layer (GCL), and they have been shown to display intrinsic phototransduction abilities, with photic properties matching those of clock entrainment [33]. The main candidate for the circadian photoreceptor is melanopsin, which is an opsin found in the eye and other photoreceptive structures in amphibians and exclusively in retinal RGCs in primates and rodents. Photic information received by RGCs is conveyed through the retinohypothalamic tract to the SCN central clock in mammals [33, 34].

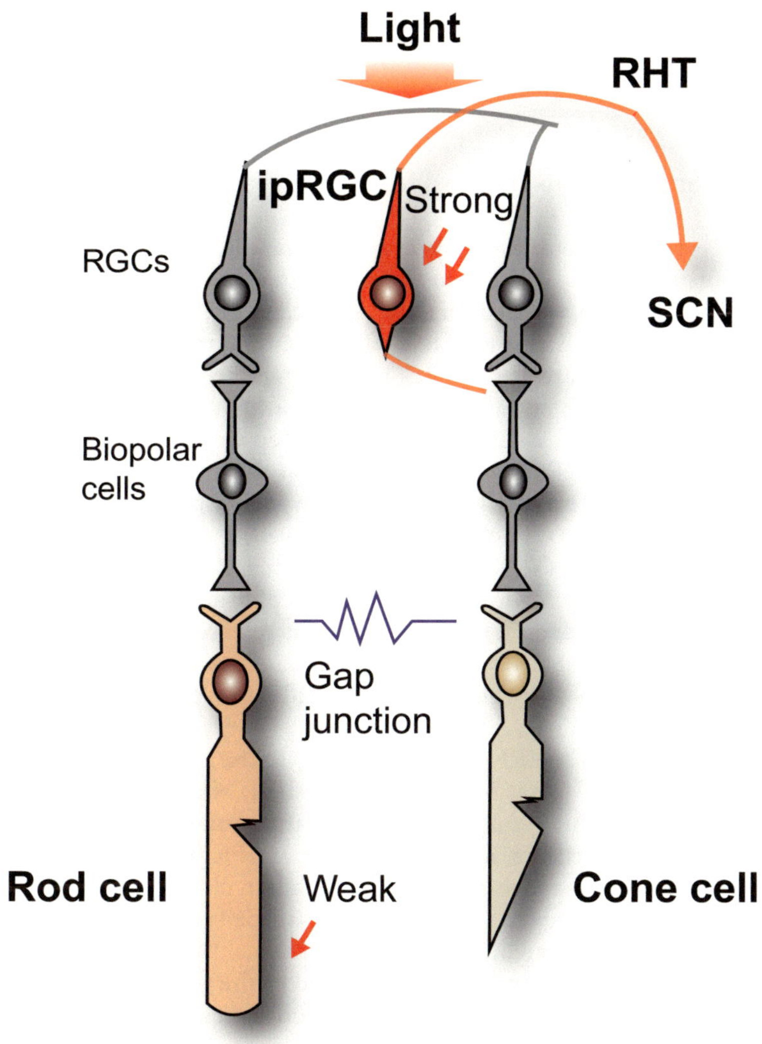

Figure 1.
Retinal cells responsible for vision and photoreception for circadian clock regulation.

4. Light-dependent transcription in the mammalian retina

Dopamine is the major catecholamine in the vertebrate retina and plays a central role in neural adaptation to light. Indeed, light stimulates the synthesis, turnover, and release of retinal dopamine, which makes dopamine an important mediator of light signaling to retinal cellular clocks [35–37]. Among the members of the dopamine-receptor family, the dopamine D2 receptor (D2R) has been shown to control light-induced reset of the circadian clock in the mouse retina [38–40]. At the molecular level, it has been reported that signaling mediated by the D2R enhances the transcriptional capacity of the CLOCK:BMAL complex. This effect involves the extracellular signal-regulated kinase (ERK)/MAPK transduction cascade and is associated with a D2R-induced increase in phosphorylation of the transcriptional coactivator, cAMP-responsive element-binding protein (CREB) and its recruitment to the CLOCK:BMAL complex [40]. Importantly, this activation of CLOCK:BMAL1-dependent transcription is responsible for the induction of the *Per1* gene by light in the retina, which is in turn responsible for the reset of the retinal cellular clock. These findings provide evidence for the physiological links among the ERK/MAPK signaling pathway, dopamine, and the light input pathway of circadian clocks.

5. Light-dependent transcription in mammalian SCN

Light resets the circadian clock by its phase-shifting properties. In particular, the phase-shifting effects of light only occur during the nighttime period of the circadian cycle. In nocturnal mammals kept in darkness, a light pulse during the subjective night (that is, the time of day corresponding to the dark period in a normal light-dark cycle) can reset the clock by evoking changes in the SCN-controlled rhythms [41–43]. If the light pulse is given at an early point in time during the subjective night, it induces a shift in SCN-controlled rhythms to a later time (phase delay). Conversely, if the light pulse is provided at the end of the subjective night, the SCN-controlled rhythms will be shifted to an earlier position in the circadian cycle (phase advance). Photic signals perceived by the retina are conveyed to the SCN through the RHT [32]. Glutamate has been identified as the major neurotransmitter responsible for transducing the photic information to the SCN along the RHT [44] (**Figure 2**). Once glutamate is released by the SCN, it binds to N-methyl-D-aspartate (NMDA) receptors, which in turn leads to the Ca^{2+} influx, that is, finally responsible for the activation of calcium-/calmodulin-dependent protein kinase (CaMK).

The involvement of the ERK/MAPK pathway in the light-input system of the circadian clock in the SCN has been well established. Mice exposed to light pulses during their subjective night display rapid ERK upregulation (phosphorylation) in the SCN [45]. Furthermore, disruption of the MAPK pathway has been shown to block light-induced phase shifting of the circadian clock at the behavioral level [46]. This finding suggests that the ERK cascade is integrally involved in photic entrainment of mammalian circadian rhythms. Events downstream of the light-induced signaling pathway in the SCN lead to the phosphorylation of cAMP-response element-binding protein (CREB), which then stimulates expression of Per1 and Per2 genes, which contain a calcium-/cAMP-response element (CRE) in their promoters [6, 47, 48]. Although the exact mechanism by which light induces early gene expression remains to be elucidated, it has been shown that a single light pulse engenders chromatin remodeling via the phosphorylation of histone H3 at Ser10 [49].

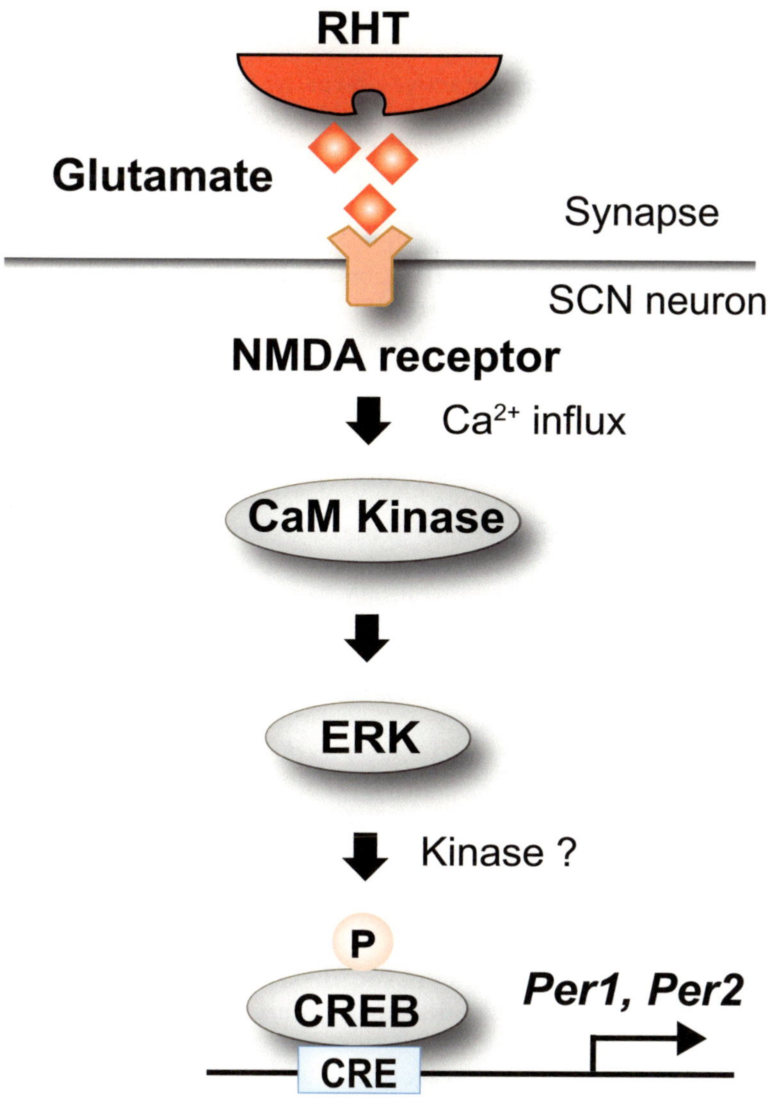

Figure 2.
Signaling cascade transducing photic signal perceived by the retina to the transcription of clock genes in SCN.

6. Light-dependent synchronization of cellular clocks in the mammalian SCN

The appropriate synchronization of cellular clocks in tissues and organs is required for the generation of circadian rhythms in a variety of physiological processes, such as sleep and metabolism [50]. In addition, the light-dependent induction of *Per1* and *Per2* is thought to contribute to the synchronization of cellular clocks in the SCN [6, 8]. However, this idea has not been fully elucidated using adequate genetically modified mice. Mouse *Per1* and *Per2* genes are induced by the CLOCK (NPAS2):BMAL complex and by light. In particular, the CLOCK (NPAS2):BMAL-dependent regulation of *Per1* and *Per2* is essential for establishment of the circadian clock's rhythmicity. Thus, genetic inhibition of both mouse *Per1* and *Per2* genes disrupts the cellular clock, preventing the analysis of synchronization [51, 52]. This problem has been solved by using zebrafish models, as described below.

7. Cellular-clock regulation in zebrafish

The zebrafish constitutes an attractive alternative to the mammalian system with which to study the complexity of circadian clock machinery and light's influence on it [9]. Characterization of the molecular components of the zebrafish circadian oscillator has revealed that the negative feedback loop in zebrafish consists of components similar to those of mammals [11]. Organ- and tissue-culture explant experiments have demonstrated that peripheral circadian oscillators are present throughout the tissues and organs of the zebrafish and that they display the remarkable feature of being light responsive [10, 13].

The characterization of components of the zebrafish cellular clock has revealed duplication of most clock genes. There are two, three, four, and eight homologues of the *Clock*, *Bmal*, *Per*, and *Cry* genes, respectively. Their circadian expression profiles and light inducibility are different, indicating the differential contribution of various clock components in the regulation of cellular clocks [28, 53–55]. For example, an investigation into the in vitro functions of the protein products of zebrafish *Cry* genes revealed that they fall into one of two groups: one group inhibits CLOCK:BMAL-mediated transcription (repressor-type CRYs: zCRY1a, zCRY1b, zCRY2a, and zCRY2b), while the other group does not inhibit transcription (non-repressor type CRYs: zCRY3, zCRY4, zCRY Dash, and plant-type zCRY).

The CLOCK (NPAS2):BMAL complex and/or light regulates the expression of zebrafish repressor types of *Crys* and *Pers* [50, 56]. The *zCry2a* and *zCry2b* genes are induced both by the CLOCK (NPAS2):BMAL complex and by light; *zCry1b*, *zPer1a*, *zPer1b*, and *zPer3* are induced by the CLOCK (NPAS2):BMAL complex but not by light; and *zCry1a* and *zPer2* are induced by light but not by the CLOCK (NPAS2):BMAL complex. These distinct dependencies of *zPer* and *zCry* gene expressions recently enabled us to uncover the role of light-induced zPER2, zCRY1a, and zCRY2a in the light-dependent synchronization of cellular clocks.

8. zPER2, zCRY1a, and zCRY2a are required for the light-dependent ontology of circadian clocks during development

In vertebrates, cellular clocks in zygotes and early embryos are not functional and become gradually set in motion during development [57, 58]. In mammals, it is quite difficult to analyze the processes of cellular-clock formation during development because embryogenesis proceeds inside the maternal uterus. Thus, the molecular mechanisms underlying the establishment of cellular clocks during vertebrate development are not well understood. Zebrafish eggs are externally fertilized and are transparent [11, 54]. In addition, zebrafish embryos develop rapidly from fertilized eggs to larvae that swim, making them an excellent model for studies investigating the ontology of vertebrate clocks.

During zebrafish development, organogenesis is completed within 2 days post-fertilization (dpf) [59]. Zebrafish larvae hatch within four dpf and start to display locomotor behavior. Zebrafish cellular clocks are autonomously set in motion during development within 1–4 dpf but are out of phase with each other in tissues and organs. Light synchronizes the phases of the cellular clocks to establish behavioral rhythms [50, 60]. Our recent study generated $zCry1a^{-/-}$ $zPer2^{-/-}$ $zCry2a^{-/-}$ triple knockout (TKO) zebrafish and used these TKO animals to show that light-induced zPER2, zCRY1a, and zCRY2a help to synchronize cellular clocks in early embryos and larvae in a light-dependent manner, thus contributing to behavioral rhythm formation in zebrafish larva [50]. Notably, these findings provide evidence that light-dependent-induced PER1 and PER2 contribute to the synchronization of cellular clocks in the SCN of mammals.

9. Light signaling pathway regulating cellular clocks in zebrafish cells

Studies using cultured zebrafish cells have identified cellular signaling cascades involved in the light-dependent regulation of cellular clocks. In several organisms, external stimuli are connected to a cell's nucleus via MAPK signaling pathways [61]. There are three major MAPKs: c-JUN N-terminal kinase (JNK), p38, and ERK. Light has been reported to activate these signaling cascades in zebrafish cells. Using a pharmacological approach, it was established that light-induced *zPer2* transactivation requires the ERK signaling pathway [15]. It has also been proposed that light-induced ERK activation triggers *zCry1a* transcription, whereas light-induced p38 activation suppresses it, highlighting a MAPK-mediated cross-regulatory mechanism for the expression of circadian-clock genes [21]. As mentioned above, evidence strongly suggests the involvement of the ERK pathway in the light-input system of the mammalian circadian clock. Thus, these findings are consistent with the idea that several aspects of the complex mammalian photo-signal transduction pathway involved in the regulation of circadian clocks are more easily investigated, both pharmacologically and molecularly, using cultured zebrafish cells. In addition, it was reported that the light-activated JNK signaling pathway induces expression of *zCry1a* and *zPer2* [62]. Notably, in contrast to these studies, it has recently been reported that the light-activated p38 pathway facilitates the expression of *zCry1a* and *zPer2* and that the ERK/MAPK signaling pathway is not involved in the light-induced expression of *zCry1a* and *zPer2* [62, 63]. The reason for these contradictory results is unknown.

10. Role of redox signaling in cellular-clock regulation by light in zebrafish

It has been proposed that the light-dependent transcription of *zCry1a* and *zPer2* is controlled through the production and removal of cellular reactive oxygen species (ROS) [16]. ROS were originally thought to act solely as toxic metabolites, because they react with components of DNA, proteins, and lipids and exert oxidative stress [64]. However, ROS are also ideally suited to be signaling molecules because they are small and can easily diffuse over short distances within a cell. In addition, mechanisms for ROS production and their rapid removal (for example, via catalase) are present in almost all cell types [64, 65]. In various organisms, light induces ROS production, which leads to an altered redox status in cells [28]. In zebrafish cells, this light-induced redox change transduces photic signals and leads to the transactivation of *zCry1a* and *zPer2* [16, 62, 66]. Importantly, light increases intracellular catalase activity by increasing the expression of *catalase*, an event that occurs after the maximum expression of the *zCry1a* and *zPer2* genes has been reached [16]. This increased catalase activity diminishes light-induced cellular ROS levels, resulting in decreased expression of the *zCry1a* and *zPer2* genes.

The toxic effects of oxidative stress have been linked to cellular ROS production induced by light-activated flavin-containing oxidases [67]. The absorbance of light in the near violet-blue region by these enzymes activates them and induces photoreduction of the flavin adenine dinucleotide (FAD) moiety, leading to ROS production. Accordingly, signaling by flavoproteins frequently induces a change in

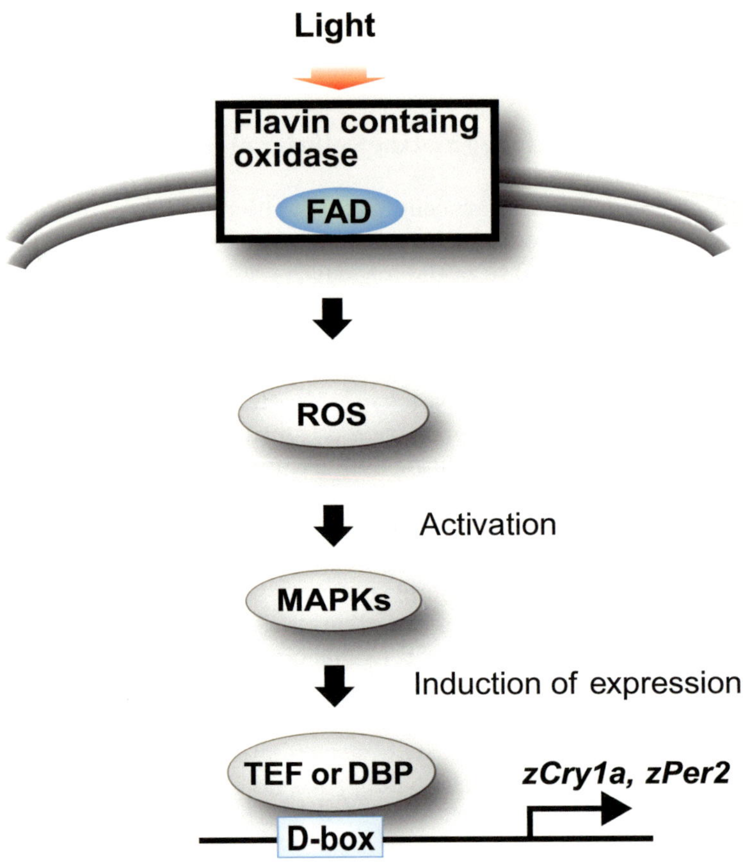

Figure 3.
Light signaling pathway regulating clock gene induction in zebrafish.

the redox state of cells [67]. Recent studies have provided evidence that flavin-containing oxidases are responsible for the light-dependent production of ROS that are second messengers coupling photoreception to photoreactivation and the circadian clock in zebrafish [62, 66] (**Figure 3**).

11. Link between circadian clocks and light-dependent DNA repair in zebrafish

Solar radiation has both beneficial and harmful effects for most species. Beneficial aspects include its role in photosynthesis and the entrainment of circadian clocks [28]. However, the UV component of solar radiation can produce cytotoxic, mutagenic, and carcinogenic lesions in DNA, which can transform or kill cells. In particular, the UV component of solar radiation produces cytotoxic and mutagenic lesions in DNA called cyclobutane pyrimidine dimers (CPDs) and pyrimidine [6-4] pyrimidone photoproducts. Photoreactivation is a light-dependent DNA repair mechanism mediated by DNA photolyases (PHRs), which bind to and repair UV-induced DNA damage using visible light as an energy source [43, 68]. Two classes of PHRs have been identified, one specific for CPDs (CPD PHRs) and the other specific for [6-4] photoproducts (64PHRs). Importantly, both the induction of PHRs in response to light and the subsequent light-dependent repair of DNA by PHRs are essential for successful photoreactivation in zebrafish cells [21]. Notably, the expression level of the *z64Phr* gene is regulated by the same light-induced MAPK cascades as those controlling the expression of the clock gene *zCry1a*, which is associated with the light-dependent regulation of the circadian clock [21, 66]. Light-induced ERK activation triggers the expression of *z64Phr*, whereas light-induced p38 activation inhibits it. Thus, both light-dependent DNA repair and regulation of the circadian clock are governed by shared regulatory pathways. Both CRYs and PHRs belong to the DNA photolyase/cryptochrome protein family and have highly similar amino acid sequences [43, 68]. Evolutionary studies have shown that the animal CRY protein functionally diverged first from the CPD photolyase and then further to generate 64PHR [69]. These facts, together with the observation that *zCry1a* and *z64Phr* share regulatory pathways, strongly indicate an evolutionary link between the circadian clock and DNA repair.

12. Conclusion

In mammals, light signals are received by the retina and then integrated with the SCN cellular clocks [7]. The SCN cellular clocks then transmit light information to peripheral cellular clocks via humoral signals and synchronize them. Recent studies have reported that factors other than cellular clocks in the SCN can synchronize peripheral cellular clocks in a light-dependent manner [42]. In contrast, in zebrafish, light directly synchronizes peripheral cellular clocks in addition to central cellular clocks [9]. Despite the differences between the light-dependent regulation of peripheral cellular clocks in mammals and zebrafish, both require similar MAPK signaling pathways and light induction of clock genes to regulate cellular clocks in a light-dependent manner.

The development of circadian clocks would be one way to segregate daytime from nighttime processes, with light-dark cycles acting as selective pressures [28]. In this scenario, increasing levels of oxygen free radicals during the daytime may have been a decisive factor in relegating the anabolic processes of mitosis, growth, and consolidation to the dark hours. Thus, it is reasonable to propose that redox signaling and stress responding pathways such as MAPKs are utilized in the light-dependent regulation of the circadian clock.

Acknowledgements

This work was supported in part by a Japan Society for the Promotion of Science (JSPS) Grant-in-Aid for Scientific Research [19K12900 (J.I.) and 18KT0068 (J.H.)]. This work was also supported by grants from the Watanabe Foundation and the Smoking Research Foundation (J.H.).

Author details

Izawa Junko[1], Yoshimi Okamoto-Uchida[2], Akari Nishimura[1] and Jun Hirayama[1]*

1 Department of Clinical Engineering, Faculty of Health Sciences, Komatsu University, Ishikawa, Japan

2 Division of Medicinal Safety Science, National Institute of Health Sciences, Tokyo, Japan

*Address all correspondence to: jun.hirayama@komatsu-u.ac.jp

References

[1] Takahashi JS. Transcriptional architecture of the mammalian circadian clock. Nature Reviews. Genetics. 2017;**18**:164-179

[2] Dunlap JC. Molecular bases for circadian clocks. Cell. 1999;**96**:271-290

[3] Hirayama J, Sassone-Corsi P. Structural and functional features of transcription factors controlling the circadian clock. Current Opinion in Genetics & Development. 2005;**15**:548-556

[4] Schibler U, Sassone-Corsi P. A web of circadian pacemakers. Cell. 2002;**111**:919-922

[5] Okamura H. Clock genes in cell clocks: Roles, actions, and mysteries. Journal of Biological Rhythms. 2004;**19**:388-399

[6] Shigeyoshi Y, Taguchi K, Yamamoto S, Takekida S, Yan L, Tei H, et al. Light-induced resetting of a mammalian circadian clock is associated with rapid induction of the mPer1 transcript. Cell. 1997;**91**:1043-1053

[7] Paul KN, Saafir TB, Tosini G. The role of retinal photoreceptors in the regulation of circadian rhythms. Reviews in Endocrine & Metabolic Disorders. 2009;**10**:271-278

[8] Okamura H, Miyake S, Sumi Y, Yamaguchi S, Yasui A, Muijtjens M, et al. Photic induction of mPer1 and mPer2 in cry-deficient mice lacking a biological clock. Science. 1999;**286**:2531-2534

[9] Tamai TK, Carr AJ, Whitmore D. Zebrafish circadian clocks: Cells that see light. Biochemical Society Transactions. 2005;**33**:962-966

[10] Whitmore D, Foulkes NS, Strahle U, Sassone-Corsi P. Zebrafish clock rhythmic expression reveals independent peripheral circadian oscillators. Nature Neuroscience. 1998;**1**:701-707

[11] Idda ML, Bertolucci C, Vallone D, Gothilf Y, Sanchez-Vazquez FJ, Foulkes NS. Circadian clocks: Lessons from fish. Progress in Brain Research. 2012;**199**:41-57

[12] Pando MP, Pinchak AB, Cermakian N, Sassone-Corsi P. A cell-based system that recapitulates the dynamic light-dependent regulation of the vertebrate clock. Proceedings of the National Academy of Sciences of the United States of America. 2001;**98**:10178-10183

[13] Whitmore D, Foulkes NS, Sassone-Corsi P. Light acts directly on organs and cells in culture to set the vertebrate circadian clock. Nature. 2000;**404**:87-91

[14] Ben-Moshe Z, Alon S, Mracek P, Faigenbloom L, Tovin A, Vatine GD, et al. The light-induced transcriptome of the zebrafish pineal gland reveals complex regulation of the circadian clockwork by light. Nucleic Acids Research. 2014;**42**:3750-3767

[15] Cermakian N, Pando MP, Thompson CL, Pinchak AB, Selby CP, Gutierrez L, et al. Light induction of a vertebrate clock gene involves signaling through blue-light receptors and MAP kinases. Current Biology: CB. 2002;**12**:844-848

[16] Hirayama J, Cho S, Sassone-Corsi P. Circadian control by the reduction/oxidation pathway: Catalase represses light-dependent clock gene expression in the zebrafish. Proceedings of the National Academy of Sciences of the United States of America. 2007;**104**:15747-15752

[17] Vallone D, Gondi SB, Whitmore D, Foulkes NS. E-box function in a period gene repressed by light. Proceedings

of the National Academy of Sciences of the United States of America. 2004;**101**:4106-4111

[18] Vatine G, Vallone D, Appelbaum L, Mracek P, Ben-Moshe Z, Lahiri K, et al. Light directs zebrafish period 2 expression via conserved D and E boxes. PLoS Biology. 2009;**7**:e1000223

[19] Dekens MP, Santoriello C, Vallone D, Grassi G, Whitmore D, Foulkes NS. Light regulates the cell cycle in zebrafish. Current Biology: CB. 2003;**13**:2051-2057

[20] Dickmeis T, Lahiri K, Nica G, Vallone D, Santoriello C, Neumann CJ, et al. Glucocorticoids play a key role in circadian cell cycle rhythms. PLoS Biology. 2007;**5**:e78

[21] Hirayama J, Miyamura N, Uchida Y, Asaoka Y, Honda R, Sawanobori K, et al. Common light signaling pathways controlling DNA repair and circadian clock entrainment in zebrafish. Cell Cycle. 2009;**8**:2794-2801

[22] Laranjeiro R, Tamai TK, Peyric E, Krusche P, Ott S, Whitmore D. Cyclin-dependent kinase inhibitor p20 controls circadian cell-cycle timing. Proceedings of the National Academy of Sciences of the United States of America. 2013;**110**:6835-6840

[23] Zhao H, Di Mauro G, Lungu-Mitea S, Negrini P, Guarino AM, Frigato E, et al. Modulation of DNA repair systems in blind cavefish during evolution in constant darkness. Current Biology: CB. 2018;**28**:3229-3243.e4

[24] King DP, Takahashi JS. Molecular genetics of circadian rhythms in mammals. Annual Review of Neuroscience. 2000;**23**:713-742

[25] Sahar S, Sassone-Corsi P. Metabolism and cancer: The circadian clock connection. Nature Reviews. Cancer. 2009;**9**:886-896

[26] Gallego M, Virshup DM. Post-translational modifications regulate the ticking of the circadian clock. Nature Reviews. Molecular Cell Biology. 2007;**8**:139-148

[27] Grimaldi B, Nakahata Y, Kaluzova M, Masubuchi S, Sassone-Corsi P. Chromatin remodeling, metabolism and circadian clocks: The interplay of CLOCK and SIRT1. The International Journal of Biochemistry & Cell Biology. 2009;**41**:81-86

[28] Uchida Y, Hirayama J, Nishina H. A common origin: Signaling similarities in the regulation of the circadian clock and DNA damage responses. Biological & Pharmaceutical Bulletin. 2010;**33**:535-544

[29] Lee HS, Nelms JL, Nguyen M, Silver R, Lehman MN. The eye is necessary for a circadian rhythm in the suprachiasmatic nucleus. Nature Neuroscience. 2003;**6**:111-112

[30] Pando MP, Sassone-Corsi P. Signaling to the mammalian circadian clocks: In pursuit of the primary mammalian circadian photoreceptor. Science's STKE. 2001;**2001**:RE16

[31] Selby CP, Thompson C, Schmitz TM, Van Gelder RN, Sancar A. Functional redundancy of cryptochromes and classical photoreceptors for nonvisual ocular photoreception in mice. Proceedings of the National Academy of Sciences of the United States of America. 2000;**97**:14697-14702

[32] Gooley JJ, Lu J, Chou TC, Scammell TE, Saper CB. Melanopsin in cells of origin of the retinohypothalamic tract. Nature Neuroscience. 2001;**4**:1165

[33] Gooley JJ, Lu J, Fischer D, Saper CB. A broad role for melanopsin in nonvisual photoreception. The Journal of Neuroscience: The Official Journal

of the Society for Neuroscience. 2003;**23**:7093-7106

[34] Viney TJ, Balint K, Hillier D, Siegert S, Boldogkoi Z, Enquist LW, et al. Local retinal circuits of melanopsin-containing ganglion cells identified by transsynaptic viral tracing. Current Biology: CB. 2007;**17**:981-988

[35] Iuvone PM, Galli CL, Garrison-Gund CK, Neff NH. Light stimulates tyrosine hydroxylase activity and dopamine synthesis in retinal amacrine neurons. Science. 1978;**202**:901-902

[36] Kramer SG. Dopamine: A retinal neurotransmitter. I. Retinal uptake, storage, and light-stimulated release of H3-dopamine in vivo. Investigative Ophthalmology. 1971;**10**:438-452

[37] Nir I, Haque R, Iuvone PM. Diurnal metabolism of dopamine in the mouse retina. Brain Research. 2000;**870**:118-125

[38] Doi M, Yujnovsky I, Hirayama J, Malerba M, Tirotta E, Sassone-Corsi P, et al. Impaired light masking in dopamine D2 receptor-null mice. Nature Neuroscience. 2006;**9**:732-734

[39] Vallone D, Picetti R, Borrelli E. Structure and function of dopamine receptors. Neuroscience and Biobehavioral Reviews. 2000;**24**:125-132

[40] Yujnovsky I, Hirayama J, Doi M, Borrelli E, Sassone-Corsi P. Signaling mediated by the dopamine D2 receptor potentiates circadian regulation by CLOCK:BMAL1. Proceedings of the National Academy of Sciences of the United States of America. 2006;**103**:6386-6391

[41] Dibner C, Schibler U, Albrecht U. The mammalian circadian timing system: Organization and coordination of central and peripheral clocks. Annual Review of Physiology. 2010;**72**:517-549

[42] Husse J, Eichele G, Oster H. Synchronization of the mammalian circadian timing system: Light can control peripheral clocks independently of the SCN clock: Alternate routes of entrainment optimize the alignment of the body's circadian clock network with external time. Bio essays: News and reviews in molecular, cellular and. Developmental Biology. 2015;**37**:1119-1128

[43] Sancar A. Cryptochrome: The second photoactive pigment in the eye and its role in circadian photoreception. Annual Review of Biochemistry. 2000;**69**:31-67

[44] Albers HE, Walton JC, Gamble KL, McNeill JK, Hummer DL. The dynamics of GABA signaling: Revelations from the circadian pacemaker in the suprachiasmatic nucleus. Frontiers in Neuroendocrinology. 2017;**44**:35-82

[45] Obrietan K, Impey S, Storm DR. Light and circadian rhythmicity regulate MAP kinase activation in the suprachiasmatic nuclei. Nature Neuroscience. 1998;**1**:693-700

[46] Antoun G, Bouchard-Cannon P, Cheng HY. Regulation of MAPK/ERK signaling and photic entrainment of the suprachiasmatic nucleus circadian clock by Raf kinase inhibitor protein. The Journal of Neuroscience: The Official Journal of the Society for Neuroscience. 2012;**32**:4867-4877

[47] Serchov T, Heumann R. Ras activity tunes the period and modulates the entrainment of the Suprachiasmatic clock. Frontiers in Neurology. 2017;**8**:264

[48] Travnickova-Bendova Z, Cermakian N, Reppert SM, Sassone-Corsi P. Bimodal regulation of mPeriod promoters by CREB-dependent signaling and CLOCK/BMAL1 activity. Proceedings of the National Academy

of Sciences of the United States of America. 2002;**99**:7728-7733

[49] Crosio C, Cermakian N, Allis CD, Sassone-Corsi P. Light induces chromatin modification in cells of the mammalian circadian clock. Nature Neuroscience. 2000;**3**:1241-1247

[50] Hirayama J, Alifu Y, Hamabe R, Yamaguchi S, Tomita J, Maruyama Y, et al. The clock components period 2, Cryptochrome 1a, and Cryptochrome 2a function in establishing light-dependent behavioral rhythms and/or total activity levels in zebrafish. Scientific Reports. 2019;**9**:196

[51] Bae K, Jin X, Maywood ES, Hastings MH, Reppert SM, Weaver DR. Differential functions of mPer1, mPer2, and mPer3 in the SCN circadian clock. Neuron. 2001;**30**:525-536

[52] Zheng B, Albrecht U, Kaasik K, Sage M, Lu W, Vaishnav S, et al. Nonredundant roles of the mPer1 and mPer2 genes in the mammalian circadian clock. Cell. 2001;**105**:683-694

[53] Daiyasu H, Ishikawa T, Kuma K, Iwai S, Todo T, Toh H. Identification of cryptochrome DASH from vertebrates. Genes to Cells. 2004;**9**:479-495

[54] Hirayama J, Kaneko M, Cardone L, Cahill G, Sassone-Corsi P. Analysis of circadian rhythms in zebrafish. Methods in Enzymology. 2005;**393**:186-204

[55] Vatine G, Vallone D, Gothilf Y, Foulkes NS. It's time to swim! Zebrafish and the circadian clock. FEBS Letters. 2011;**585**:1485-1494

[56] Kobayashi Y, Ishikawa T, Hirayama J, Daiyasu H, Kanai S, Toh H, et al. Molecular analysis of zebrafish photolyase/cryptochrome family: Two types of cryptochromes present in zebrafish. Genes to Cells. 2000;**5**:725-738

[57] Dekens MP, Whitmore D. Autonomous onset of the circadian clock in the zebrafish embryo. The EMBO Journal. 2008;**27**:2757-2765

[58] Kaneko M, Cahill GM. Light-dependent development of circadian gene expression in transgenic zebrafish. PLoS Biology. 2005;**3**:e34

[59] Cahill GM. Clock mechanisms in zebrafish. Cell and Tissue Research. 2002;**309**:27-34

[60] Kazimi N, Cahill GM. Development of a circadian melatonin rhythm in embryonic zebrafish. Brain Research. Developmental Brain Research. 1999;**117**:47-52

[61] Thomas GM, Huganir RL. MAPK cascade signalling and synaptic plasticity. Nature Reviews. Neuroscience. 2004;**5**:173-183

[62] Pagano C, Siauciunaite R, Idda ML, Ruggiero G, Ceinos RM, Pagano M, et al. Evolution shapes the responsiveness of the D-box enhancer element to light and reactive oxygen species in vertebrates. Scientific Reports. 2018;**8**:13180

[63] Mracek P, Santoriello C, Idda ML, Pagano C, Ben-Moshe Z, Gothilf Y, et al. Regulation of per and cry genes reveals a central role for the D-box enhancer in light-dependent gene expression. PLoS One. 2012;**7**:e51278

[64] Neill SJ, Desikan R, Clarke A, Hurst RD, Hancock JT. Hydrogen peroxide and nitric oxide as signalling molecules in plants. Journal of Experimental Botany. 2002b;**53**:1237-1247

[65] Neill S, Desikan R, Hancock J. Hydrogen peroxide signalling. Current Opinion in Plant Biology. 2002a;**5**:388-395

[66] Osaki T, Uchida Y, Hirayama J, Nishina H. Diphenyleneiodonium

chloride, an inhibitor of reduced nicotinamide adenine dinucleotide phosphate oxidase, suppresses light-dependent induction of clock and DNA repair genes in zebrafish. Biological & Pharmaceutical Bulletin. 2011;**34**:1343-1347

[67] Hockberger PE, Skimina TA, Centonze VE, Lavin C, Chu S, Dadras S, et al. Activation of flavin-containing oxidases underlies light-induced production of H_2O_2 in mammalian cells. Proceedings of the National Academy of Sciences of the United States of America. 1999;**96**:6255-6260

[68] Todo T. Functional diversity of the DNA photolyase/blue light receptor family. Mutation Research. 1999;**434**:89-97

[69] Cashmore AR, Jarillo JA, Wu YJ, Liu D. Cryptochromes: Blue light receptors for plants and animals. Science. 1999;**284**:760-765

Section 3

Chronobiology of the Cardiovascular System

Chapter 4

Circadian Rhythm of Blood Pressure in Children and Adolescents

Anastasiia Ledyaeva, Sergey Klauchek and Mikhail Ledyaev

Abstract

Everything in our body is under control of central and peripheral pacemakers that regulate all the processes and functions according to the day-night and sleep-wake cycles. Cardiovascular system is not an exception. Blood pressure, heart rate, and even vascular resistance have circadian patterns. Nowadays new diagnostic devices provide all necessary data on 24-h variation of the hemodynamic parameters in patients of all ages. Due to the complex regulation mechanisms which underline this variation, circadian patterns are not the same in different people. Why do we need to assess these rhythms? First of all, it is a key to the early diagnosis of different cardiovascular diseases and their complications. When the circadian rhythm is impaired, for example, the level of blood pressure is within the normal ranges, but it does not decline at night or even is higher than at daytime, there is an increased risk of the development of arterial hypertension and target organ damage. There is a large amount of studies on 24-h rhythm of blood pressure in adults. On the contrary, in children there is still a lack of data on this topic.

Keywords: circadian rhythm, blood pressure, adolescence, circadian index, ambulatory blood pressure monitoring

1. Introduction

All physiological processes in the organism have a cyclic organization—from thermoregulation and activity of cardiovascular system (CVS) and respiratory systems to expression of genes, mitochondrial activity, and synthesis of proteins [1–3]. Endogenous rhythms in newborns are formed under the impact of exogenous synchronizers, such as light and sound. Circadian organization of excretion with urine of sodium and potassium occurs in a period from the 4th till the 20th week; on 2–3 weeks of the postnatal development, the synchronization of a body temperature with the day-night cycle takes place. At the present time, the active development of biomedical technologies allows to register and analyze the circadian variability of blood pressure (BP), heart rate (HR), and heart rate variability (HRV) by conducting their monitoring during 24 and more hours. The interest of scientists and clinical physicians to the diurnal variabilities of CVS parameters is also connected with the fact that based on the condition of the biological rhythms of a separate system of organs it is possible to judge the functional condition of an organism, the level of its adaptive opportunities, the risks of development of cardiovascular diseases, and even about the activity of pathological process [4–6].

In the circadian pattern of BP, two peaks are allocated: the first one is registered in the morning, from 6 to 12 a.m., the second one, smaller in amplitude, at about 7 h p.m. Circadian rhythm of BP is determined by numerous exogenous (light, noise, temperature, and eating behavior) and endogenous (melatonin, sympathetic tone, renin-angiotensin-aldosterone system (RAAS), NO and endothelin-1 level, etc.) factors [7, 8].

The group of pacemakers, forming the suprachiasmatic nucleus of hypothalamus (SCN), located directly above the optic chiasm, is a central pacer of circadian rhythms, synchronized with the sleep-waking cycle. SCN mediates the secretion of corticoids that in turn increase the sensitivity of vascular wall to the catecholamines and decrease the production of vasodilators [9]. Peripheral clock genes (Per1, Bmal1, Cry1, and Cry2) control the sensitivity of α-adrenoreceptors to vasoconstrictors [10].

Melatonin is a hormone of pineal gland that stays in the core of our sleep behavior. Regulation of melatonin secretion is controlled by light through the retinothalamic track and suprachiasmatic nucleus of hypothalamus. At the same time, it is an important vasoactive factor, and thus it forms the circadian BP profile [11, 12]. Also it regulates the synthesis of catecholamines by adrenals and mediates the sensitivity of baroreflex [13, 14]. The concentration of melatonin in plasma and 6-sulfaoxymelatonin in urea is decreased in non-dippers [15, 16]. The administration of melatonin in patients with hypertension leads to the decrease of the average values of SBP and DBP without change of sleep behavior [17]. It is interesting that melatonin has two faces: he could be a vasoconstrictor or vasodilator [18]. It is so because there are two types of melatonin receptors: MT1 and MT2. Low melatonin concentrations activate MT1 receptors and lead to vasoconstriction. In high concentration, melatonin provides an opposite effect through the stimulation of MT2 receptors [19].

Angiotensin 2 is another powerful oscillator of 24-h dynamic of BP. The peak of activity of renin in plasma and concentration of angiotensin-2 relate to early morning, explaining the morning rise of BP [20]. Thus, the combined influence of exogenic and endogenic oscillators forms the normal circadian rhythm of BP, providing an adequate blood supply of organs and tissues, depending on requirements of an organism.

In healthy humans there is a BP decline by 10–20% and rapid increase of BP in the early morning hours [21]. Circadian BP pattern can be assessed during ABPM by calculation of circadian index (CI)—the main characteristic of the nocturnal BP reduction. CI is a percent decline in mean BP during sleep relative to the mean BP during daytime wakefulness. CI is calculated as ((awake BP mean − asleep BP mean)/awake BP mean) × 100. Due to the value of CI, there are four types of circadian BP patterns: "dipper" 10–20%, "non-dipper" 0–10%, "overdipper" >20%, and "night-peaker" or "riser" with nocturnal increase of BP—CI being negative.

A change of the internal structure of circadian rhythm of BP is followed by the shift of acrophase at a later time and the decrease of BP variability. There is the definite genetic aptitude to change of the daily BP profile. The optimal degree of an overnight decrease is characterized by the presence of allele D, genotype DD gene ACE, and genotype 4a/4b gene of the endothelial synthase of a nitrogen oxide. While insufficient overnight BP decrease is associated with the presence of allele I, genotype II, and genotype 4b/4b gene of this enzyme, as well as the different types of reactivity of the vegetative nervous system.

Misalignment and change of the structure of biorhythms are not independent pathology. It is considered as a prenosological condition that reflects an impaired system of regulation of physiological functions and the risk of development of cardiovascular diseases [4].

2. Circadian rhythms of peripheral (brachial) and central (aortic) blood pressure in adolescents

The main problem in pediatrics is that new approaches that are developed in medical diagnostics are firstly probated in adults, and it takes sometimes years before they will be approved for usage in children. The ambulatory blood pressure monitoring is not the exception. There are several studies that make a fundament for the guidelines and show the important role of that method in early diagnostic of arterial hypertension (AH) in young population, but it seems that the normal ranges of some chronobiological parameters were taken from adults' guidelines without any changes. But we have to keep in mind that adolescents could have some peculiarities of circadian organization of different biological parameters due to changes in hormonal regulation that follow the puberty. This hypothesis is based also on the data published by some authors. For example, it seems interesting why overdipping pattern for DBP is so common and is not so for SBP.

Due to a lack of data on peculiarities of circadian patterns in adolescents, we performed a study in 354 healthy children from 12 to 17 years old. The average nocturnal BP decline did not differ in boys and girls ($p > 0.05$). Average CI for brachial systolic BP was 12.2%; for brachial diastolic BP, 18.3%; and for brachial mean BP, 15.5%. Average CI for aortic systolic BP was 12%; for aortic diastolic BP, 19.5%; and for aortic mean BP, 16%.

Then we looked at the distribution of different circadian BP profiles in the studied group. The majority (71.8%) of adolescents were "dippers" for SBP, 26.5% were "non-dippers" for SBP, and the minority (1.7%) of adolescents were "overdippers" for SBP (**Figure 1**). In the case of DPB, there were different results: 50.3% "dippers," 10.5% "non-dippers," and 39.3% "overdippers" (**Figure 2**).

The results of descriptive statistics of CI of brachial BP are shown in **Table 1** (girls) and **Table 2** (boys). Our findings supported the hypothesis that the normal ranges for CI in children differ from ranges for adults. The data from percentile rank could be interpreted in the following way: 25–75 percentile is the normal range, 5–25 percentile shows the values of the parameter that are lower than normal, 75–95 percentile is the values that are higher than normal, and <5 percentile and >95% provide the lowest and the highest values that in clinical practice describe the pathological change in the parameter. The normal range for CI of SBP in adolescents

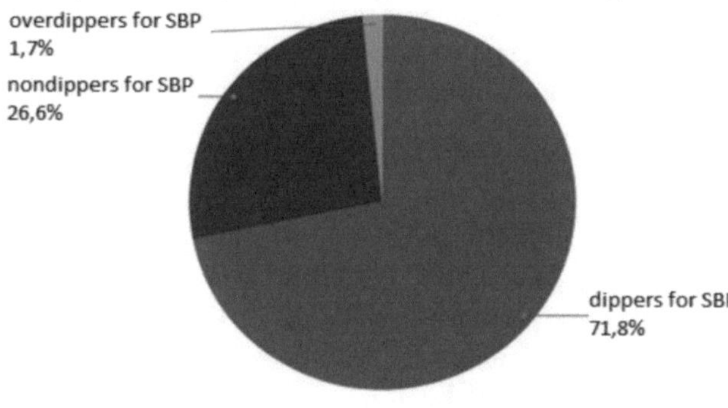

Figure 1.
The distribution of different circadian SBP profiles in the studied group.

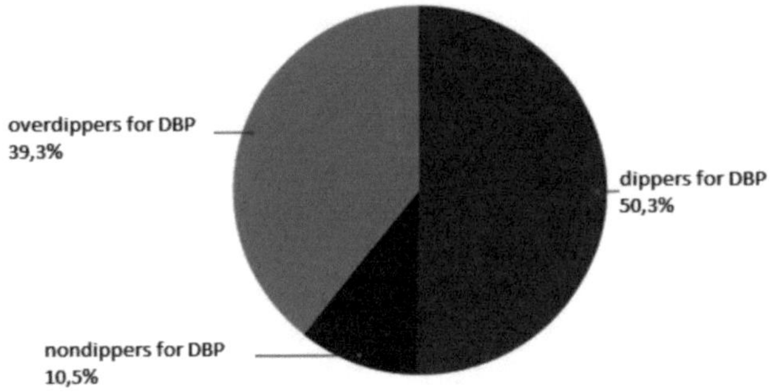

Figure 2.
The distribution of different circadian DBP profiles in the studied group.

Parameter	Mean	Minimum	Median	Maximum	Percentile			
					5	25	75	95
CI SBP (%)	12.1	0	12	26	5	9	15	19
CI DBP (%)	18.2	1	18.5	33	6.3	14	23	28
CI MBP (%)	15.8	2	16	28	6	12	19.5	24

Table 1.
Descriptive statistics of circadian index of brachial BP and its percentile distribution in adolescent girls.

Parameter	Mean	Minimum	Median	Maximum	Percentile			
					5	25	75	95
CI SBP (%)	12.14	1	12	24	5	9	15	19
CI DBP (%)	18.29	2	18	34	7	14	23	29
CI MBP (%)	15.19	3	15	38	6	12	19	24

Table 2.
Descriptive statistics of circadian index and its percentile distribution in adolescent boys.

is 9–15%, for CI of DBP is 14–23%, and for CI of MBP is 12–20%. Thereby for DBP the nocturnal dipping has a greater extend in physiological conditions in comparison with the SBP. This supported by statistical analysis that showed the significant differences in average values 12.1% (CI SBP) versus 18.2 (CI DBP) ($p < 0.05$) in adolescents of both sexes. As shown above, we talk about impaired circadian BP profile in adults using the same normal ranges for SBP and DBP<10% and higher than 20% of nocturnal decline of BP. But in children we found different values: the impaired SBP circadian profile is <5% and higher than 19%, DBP profile <6 and >28%, and MBP profile <6 and >24%. So, one can see that the profile "overdipping" for DBP starts from higher values in children in comparison with adults.

There was similar data for CI of aortic BP (**Table 3** for girls, **Table 4** for boys). Aortic DBP decrease to the greater extend at night in comparison with aortic SBP and MBP ($p < 0.05$).

In adolescents with dipping daily profile of SBP and DBP (a nocturnal decrease from 10 to 20%), the relative power of LF% during day was 35.1 ± 1.1%, LF% at night was 27.1 ± 1.8%, HF% during day was 28.3 ± 2.1%, HF% at night was 35.2 ± 1.9%, and circadian index of LF/HF was 1.3 ± 0.007, showing the physiological daily rhythm of fluctuations in the ratio between sympathetic and parasympathetic regulation contour.

In adolescents the degree of nighttime decline in the SBP exceeded 20%, the relative power of LF% during wakefulness was significantly higher than in adolescents with a normal decrease in the SBP at night (41.2 ± 1.7 vs. 35.1 ± 1, 1%, respectively, $p < 0.05$), and the circadian index of LF/HF was 1.5 ± 0.006. In adolescents with an excessive decrease in DBP, the circadian index LF/HF was 1.7 ± 0.006, and the relative power of LF and VLF% during the day was significantly higher in comparison with adolescents with a normal decrease in DBP (42.6 ± 2.1% against 35.1 ± 1.1% for LF%; 33.7 ± 1.1 vs. 27.2 ± 2.1% for VLF%, $p < 0.05$).

In adolescents with insufficient nighttime decreases in SBP and/or DBP (<10%), the circadian index LF/HF was 1.1 ± 0.007, which indicates a relative absence of a change in the ratio of the parasympathetic and sympathetic regulations at night and, as a result, smaller amplitude of the circadian rhythm of the activity of the autonomic nervous system. The average values of the relative power of LF and HF% in the group with an insufficient decrease in SBP and/or DBP during wakefulness did not significantly differ from the group with normal nocturnal decline in BP ($p > 0.05$). The main characteristic of this group of adolescents was the absence of a significant decrease in the relative power of LF% at night (37.1 ± 2.1% during the day vs. 32.2 ± 1.9% at night).

Puberty is a difficult critical period of the development, and every age in that period has its peculiarities. We performed ANOVA with post hoc Bonferroni test to find out if there are any differences in CI of CBP, DBP, and MBP in three age subgroups: 12–13, 14–15, and 16–17 years. The results are shown in **Table 5** (for brachial BP in boys), **Table 6** (for brachial BP in girls), **Table 7** (for aortic BP in boys), and **Table 8** (for aortic BP in girls). In boys there was a significant difference in the value of CI SBP and CI DBP between boys of different age subgroups ($p < 0.05$). That was supported by the results of Pearson correlation analysis between the CI and age, but the link is weak, so even if it is significant ($p < 0.05$), the hypothesis that the value of CI decreases with age has to be approved in the future studies. In girls, there were neither significant difference in the value of CI between age subgroups nor a significant correlation between CI and age ($p > 0.05$). We suppose that this can be explained by the different times of the puberty onset in boys and girls. As we know,

Parameter	Mean	Minimum	Median	Maximum	Percentile			
					5	25	75	95
CI SBP (%)	12	1	12	25	4	8	16	20
CI DBP (%)	20	3	21	42	8	15	25	31
CI MBP (%)	16	2	17	34	7	13	20	25

Table 3.
Descriptive statistics of circadian index of aortic BP and its percentile distribution in adolescent girls.

Parameter	Mean	Minimum	Median	Maximum	Percentile			
					5	25	75	95
CI SBP (%)	12	0	11	24	5	8	15	19
CI DBP (%)	19	3	19	34	6	14	24	30
CI MBP (%)	16	3	16	28	6	12	19	24

Table 4.
Descriptive statistics of circadian index of aortic BP and its percentile distribution in adolescent boys.

the main hormonal changes in girls start earlier, so by the age of 12–13, they have higher stage of puberty in comparison with boys. It is necessary to provide the same study in younger children. The main limitation of our study was that the adolescents in different age subgroups are not the same, so it was not the same boy or girl who was growing up from 12 to 17 years old. Thus, we cannot rule out other individual peculiarities of adolescent organism that could affect the results.

Parameter	12–13 years old (n = 46)	14–15 years old (n = 68)	16–17 years old (n = 56)	p-value
CI SBP (%)	13 ± 0.6	12 ± 0.5	11 ± 0.5	$p < 0.05$
CI DBP (%)	19 ± 0.9	18 ± 0.8	17 ± 0.8	$p < 0.05$
CI MBP (%)	15.9 ± 1.0	14.0 ± 0.7	15.8 ± 0.7	$p > 0.05$
r Pearson (age/CI SBP)		−0.2		$p < 0.05$
r Pearson (age/CI DBP)		−0.2		$p < 0.05$
r Pearson (age/CI MBP)		−0.1		$p > 0.05$

Table 5.
Value of circadian index of brachial BP in age subgroups of adolescent boys.

Parameter	12–13 years old (n = 52)	14–15 years old (n = 74)	16–17 years old (n = 58)	p-value
CI SBP (%)	13 ± 0.6	12 ± 0.5	12 ± 0.7	$p > 0.05$
CI DBP (%)	21 ± 0.9	18 ± 0.8	19 ± 1.0	$p > 0.05$
CI MBP (%)	16.8 ± 0.7	15.5 ± 0.6	15.4 ± 0.9	$p > 0.05$
r Pearson (age/CI SBP)		−0.01		$p > 0.05$
r Pearson (age/CI DBP)		−0.1		$p > 0.05$
r Pearson (age/CI MBP)		−0.1		$p > 0.05$

Table 6.
Value of circadian index of brachial BP in age subgroups of adolescent girls.

Parameter	12–13 years old (n = 46)	14–15 years old (n = 68)	16–17 years old (n = 56)	p-value
CI SBP (%)	13 ± 0.8	11 ± 0.5	10 ± 0.5	$p < 0.05$
CI DBP (%)	21 ± 1.0	19 ± 0.8	17 ± 0.8	$p < 0.05$
CI MBP (%)	18.3 ± 0.8	16.6 ± 0.7	15.6 ± 0.9	$p = 0.08$
r Pearson (age/CI SBP)		−0.2		$p < 0.05$
r Pearson (age/CI DBP)		−0.2		$p < 0.05$
r Pearson (age/CI MBP)		−0.2		$p > 0.05$

Table 7.
Value of circadian index of aortic BP in age subgroups of adolescent boys.

Parameter	12–13 years old ($n = 52$)	14–15 years old ($n = 74$)	16–17 years old ($n = 58$)	*p*-value
CI SBP (%)	12 ± 0.6	11 ± 0.5	11 ± 0.8	$p > 0.05$
CI DBP (%)	21 ± 0.8	19 ± 0.8	19 ± 1.0	$p > 0.05$
CI MBP (%)	17.5 ± 0.8	17.4 ± 0.7	18.1 ± 0.8	$p > 0.05$
r Pearson (age/CI SBP)		−0.04		$p > 0.05$
r Pearson (age/CI DBP)		−0.1		$p > 0.05$
r Pearson (age/CI MBP)		−0.03		$p > 0.05$

Table 8.
Value of circadian index of aortic BP in age subgroups of adolescent girls.

3. Conclusion

Analysis of the circadian rhythm of the peripheral and central blood pressure revealed gender-related features of the diurnal SBP and DBP profiles—the decrease of the degree of nocturnal decline in brachial and aortic pressure with age in healthy boys and the absence of such changes in girls 12–17 years old. The tendency to decrease with age of the degree of nocturnal dip in peripheral pressure in young men indicates the peculiarities of the age dynamics of the formation of the circadian organization of the vegetative mechanisms of regulation of the vascular wall stiffness that underlie the formation of daily arterial pressure profile. The circadian rhythm of brachial and aortic diastolic pressure in adolescents was characterized by a shift of the 25–75 percentile ranges toward higher levels of the degree of nocturnal dip in DBP compared to that for the SBP (14–23 and 9–15%, respectively). This could be probably due to the different contribution of the vasomotor component to the formation of circadian fluctuations of systolic and diastolic pressures. In addition, the values of 95 percentile, by which the disturbance of the arterial blood pressure profile is pronounced, were 28–29% for brachial and aortic diastolic pressures, which exceeds the generally accepted standard values for the adult population (22%). Thus it is necessary to provide more studies on mechanisms that underline the differences. The obtained data can be used to improve accuracy when decoding data of ABPM and interpretation of the results obtained in adolescents.

Conflict of interest

The authors declare no conflict of interest.

Author details

Anastasiia Ledyaeva*, Sergey Klauchek and Mikhail Ledyaev
Volgograd State Medical University, Volgograd, Russia

*Address all correspondence to: a.m.ledyaeva@gmail.com

References

[1] Refinetti R, Menaker M. The circadian rhythm of body temperature. Physiology & Behavior. 1992;**51**(3):613-637

[2] Spengler CM, Czeisler CA, Shea SA. An endogenous circadian rhythm of respiratory control in humans. The Journal of Physiology. 2000;**526**(3):683-694

[3] Van Dongen HPA, Kerkhof GA, Dinges DF. Human circadian rhythms. Molecular Biology of Circadian Rhythms. 2004:255-269

[4] Sato M et al. Possible contribution of chronobiology to cardiovascular health. Frontiers in Physiology. 2014;**4**:409

[5] Rios MT et al. Prognostic value of the sleep-time relative blood pressure decline in normotensive individuals: The hygia project. Journal of the American Society of Hypertension. 2015;**9**(4):9-10

[6] Turner JR, Viera AJ, Shimbo D. Ambulatory blood pressure monitoring in clinical practice: A review. The American Journal of Medicine. 2015;**128**(1):14-20

[7] Hermida RC et al. Decreasing sleep-time blood pressure determined by ambulatory monitoring reduces cardiovascular risk. Journal of the American College of Cardiology. 2011;**58**(11):1165-1173

[8] Sherwood A et al. Blood pressure dipping: Ethnicity, sleep quality, and sympathetic nervous system activity. American Journal of Hypertension. 2011;**24**(9):982-988

[9] Yang S, Zhang L. Glucocorticoids and vascular reactivity. Current Vascular Pharmacology. 2004;**2**(1):1-12

[10] Masuki S et al. Reduced α-adrenoceptor responsiveness and enhanced baroreflex sensitivity in cry-deficient mice lacking a biological clock. The Journal of Physiology. 2005;**566**(1):213-224

[11] Ekmekcioglu C. Melatonin receptors in humans: Biological role and clinical relevance. Biomedicine & Pharmacotherapy. 2006;**60**(3):97-108

[12] Peliciari-Garcia RA et al. Expression of circadian clock and melatonin receptors within cultured rat cardiomyocytes. Chronobiology International. 2011;**28**(1):21-30

[13] Kitajima T et al. The effects of oral melatonin on the autonomic function in healthy subjects. Psychiatry and Clinical Neurosciences. 2001;**55**(3):299-300

[14] Pechanova O. Impact of melatonin on central blood pressure regulation. Paulis L, Simko F. Activitas Nervosa Superior Rediviva. 2016;**58**(4):99-104

[15] Jonas M et al. Impaired nocturnal melatonin secretion in non-dipper hypertensive patients. Blood Pressure. 2003;**12**(1):19-24

[16] Zeman M et al. Plasma melatonin concentrations in hypertensive patients with the dipping and non-dipping blood pressure profile. Life Sciences. 2005;**76**(16):1795-1803

[17] Scheer FAJL, van Doornen LJP, Buijs RM. Light and diurnal cycle affect autonomic cardiac balance in human; possible role for the biological clock. Autonomic Neuroscience. 2004;**110**(1):44-48

[18] Pandi-Perumal SR et al. Physiological effects of melatonin: Role of melatonin receptors and signal transduction pathways. Progress in Neurobiology. 2008;**85**(3):335-353

[19] Tunstall RR et al. MT2 receptors mediate the inhibitory effects of

melatonin on nitric oxide-induced relaxation of porcine isolated coronary arteries. Journal of Pharmacology and Experimental Therapeutics. 2011;**336**(1):127-133

[20] Marc Y, Llorens-Cortes C. The role of the brain renin–angiotensin system in hypertension: Implications for new treatment. Progress in Neurobiology. 2011;**95**(2):89-103

[21] Smolensky MH, Hermida RC, Portaluppi F. Circadian mechanisms of 24-hour blood pressure regulation and patterning. Sleep Medicine Reviews. 2017;**33**:4-16

Section 4

Chronobiology of the Autonomic Nervous System

Chapter 5

Circadian Rhythms of the Autonomic Nervous System: Scientific Implication and Practical Implementation

Marc N. Jarczok, Harald Guendel, Jennifer J. McGrath and Elisabeth M. Balint

Abstract

Circadian rhythms are omnipresent in almost any biosignal. In this chapter, we join them with the need for practical tools for screening in preventive settings and point out heart rate variability (HRV), a measure of autonomic nervous system activity, as a chronobiologic, unspecific index of mental and physical health. We discuss methods to calculate the circadian variation of HRV measures, particularly the cosinor procedure. We present reference values for circadian variation parameters of HRV and data concerning reproducibility. Furthermore, we show data giving first evidence of HRV as a comprehensive health index by showing altered circadian variation patterns of HRV depending on mental (trait dysthymia) as well as physical (inflammatory markers) health. Finally, we present examples of disturbed chronobiology of HRV in clinical and preventive settings and its practical application in medical consultation.

Keywords: circadian variation, heart rate variability, prevention, health index, vagal activity, occupational medicine, autonomic nervous system

1. Introduction

1.1 The need for practical tools for screening in preventive settings

Circadian rhythms are omnipresent in nearly all biosignals particularly including heart rate (HR) and blood pressure [1]. Technological advances in wearables and ambulatory monitoring have made the continuous recording of real-time data highly accessible for health researchers and clinicians. Consider, 24–48 h recordings of blood pressure are frequently used in the clinical context to determine what grade of hypertension a patient has to ensure better options for treatment [2, 3]. In other areas, systematic and statistical analysis of circadian rhythms may offer adjuvant avenues such as in occupational medicine. Nonetheless, traditional approaches in this field included foremost prevention of injuries, e.g., from chemical or other environmental hazards. In the past years, the catalog of potential hazards was extended to mental health-related problems like stress and communicative problems. Moreover, the tasks in occupational medicine include now an active (occupational) health management rather than just hazard avoidance. This is mirrored by federal demands. For example, the German Federal Institute for Occupational Safety and Health (Bundesanstalt für Arbeitsschutz und Arbeitsmedizin, BAuA) just recently extended the instrument for risk assessment at the workplace ("Gefährdungsbeurteilung") [4] now covering also psychological hazards such as work stress and thus moved the field further toward the area of occupational health management. Unfortunately, these risk assessments are often based on individuals' self-report only. This is not at least due to the fact that most objective biological methods are expensive, invasive, and/or complicated. For example, assessing a full cortisol profile (a prominent stress hormone) comprising eight saliva samples during the day is accompanied by low compliance because participants perceive the strict protocol (exact timings, no food, no coffee, no cigarettes in the first hour post-awakening) as impracticable and the reliability is being blunted by violating the measurement protocol [5]. In addition, most available biomarkers have a high disease specificity, since they originated from clinically focused applications. While in the clinical context a high disease specificity of a biomarker is a major diagnostic requirement, it precludes a broad application, for example, in the occupational prevention contexts (i.e., company-wide health screenings or health checks). For example, assessing a comprehensible health check with blood count, physical tests, and ophthalmologic and audiometric examination easily adds up to several hundred euros per examination, but the resources available for health screenings are limited. One solution is the enrollment of comprehensive health check to a limited group of persons—usually higher managers. Therefore, in the given scenario of limited resources, it appears desirable to identify biomarkers which are less disease-specific but more widely and reliably able to indicate that *something* is wrong even on a preclinical stage (high sensitivity) and, in this case, direct the individual to further examinations, e.g., at the company physician. In addition, in the context of prevention, this biomarker should be easy to measure at low costs and be practicable to assess in the routine of occupational health physicians [6–8].

1.2 Heart rate variability as a measure of autonomic nervous activity: a chronobiologic, unspecific index of mental and physical health

Several attempts to find a more general health index have been previously made. For example, the Allostatic Load Index (ALI) aims to measure the bodily "wear and tear" and to identify individuals before chronic health disturbances emerge [9–11]. It represents an assessment of the cumulative burden of psychosocial factors on health by exploring alterations in different biological systems but has some limitations [6–8, 11] including (A) invasive procedures, (B) cost-intensive examination, and (C) results which are relative to the investigated population and therefore not promptly available but only after the vast majority of the population has been investigated. Other screening tools encompass risk prediction of the development of (fatal) heart diseases (events) such as Framingham, PROCAM, SCORE-CVD, or SCORE-CHD risk scores but suffer from similar issues as the ALI score since they are based on a comparable set of biomarkers. One common aim of these screening tools is the detection of dysregulation, i.e., abnormal high or low values compared to a given clinical (usually age-adjusted) reference or population distribution (percentile). The vast majority of these biomarkers can be seen as an outcome of an underlying dysregulation—at least in part. The autonomic nervous system (ANS) plays a pivotal role in adaption and homeostasis, particularly the vagus nerve. This nerve is a primary, fast, and bidirectional route conveying physiological states to the brain (sensory fibers), as well as shaping and coordinating somatic responses to adapt to environmental challenges (motor fibers) [12–15]. The central-peripheral brain-heart integration can be indexed noninvasively and inexpensively by cardiac autonomic activity using HR recordings, e.g., from chest belt HR monitors. From these HR recordings, beat-to-beat variability can be calculated (i.e., heart rate variability [HRV]), representing a valid and reliable measure of autonomic function [12, 15]. Thus, variability measures provide a window to the central autonomic nervous system (CAN). The working level of the CAN reflects the capacity of the body to adapt to environmental challenges [16] such as a problematic supervisor. It also corresponds to emotion regulation capacity [13]. Furthermore, decreased values of HRV predict premature mortality [17] and morbidity [12] such as higher inflammatory state [18–20], increased cardiovascular disease risk [21], and myocardial infarction risk [22] and have been implicated in fatigue [23], work stress [24], and pain regulation [25–28]. Latest research demonstrates associations with common mental disorders like depression [29]. Apart from diagnosed diseases, HRV shows associations with subjective measures like self-rated health [30]. Like many other biomarkers, ANS measures express a circadian variation pattern [31].

Taken together, measures of HRV seem to represent an integrative marker for mental and somatic health. Thus, these measures characterize an ideal psychosomatic marker. Promising first studies reveal short-term measures of HRV as an index of change pre- to post-therapeutic interventions [32]. However, while short-term measures (i.e., 5-minute resting baselines) are subject to situation-specific variations, long-term measures may overcome this disadvantage and additionally provide salient information from the recorded time series inherent in a 24 h signal (i.e., diurnal variation). Furthermore, the situation-related adaptability of an individual can be visualized by long-term measurements of HRV. The latter can easily be analyzed with spectral methods, shown as a comprehensive graph, and can easily be combined with diary information from a patient, making the impact of a particular situation obvious. For example, a difficult talk with a co-worker reduces the power spectrum and can be explained to the patient. Yet, the utility of long-term measures capturing the circadian variation of HRV has not been evaluated for this purpose. Still, to be further explored, circadian variation patterns of cardiac autonomic activity may present a promising candidate as an unspecific index of both overall physical and mental health.

In the following section (Section 2), we will outline how to calculate measures of circadian variation by two different methods. In Sections 3 and 4, we will present first evidence and examples of HRV as a comprehensive health index. Particularly Section 3 describes epidemiological and other research results of circadian variation patterns of cardiac autonomic activity (normal age decrements, implications in somatic and mental health disorders). In the final section (Section 4), we will present examples of disturbed chronobiology of HRV and its application in a clinical and an occupational setting as an index for health.

2. Measuring circadian variation of the ANS

While specific measures exist that represent an index of cardiac vagal activity (such as root mean square of successive differences [RMSSD], respiratory sinus arrhythmia [RSA], percentage of the NN intervals >50 ms [PNN50]), others measure index more general cardiac autonomic activity (i.e., mixed sympathetic and parasympathetic) such as the standard deviation of normal interbeat intervals (SDNN) or total power (TP). For an excellent and detailed overview of metric and norms, see, for example, [15].

Cardiac autonomic activity exhibits a pattern of diurnal variation. The circadian timing system regulates daily modulation of synchronized physiological activity in order to conserve energy expenditure and the use of internal resources, thereby optimizing functioning at the ideal time of day (i.e., coordinate physiological functions and behavior) [1, 33]. The circadian timing system is organized hierarchically by the central pacemaker within the suprachiasmatic nucleus (SCN) [1, 2]. This master pacemaker orchestrates the rhythmicity of endogenous, or self-sustained, clocks within different central and peripheral tissues, which autoregulate through transcriptional and translational feedback loops. Genetic variations in circadian locomotor output cycles kaput (CLOCK) genes are implicated in unique phenotypes, including timing of sleep preference (evening type), metabolism, and mood regulation. More generally, endogenous molecular clocks enable organisms to anticipate environmental challenges. These endogenous pacemakers are also entrained by environmental context, including cyclical changes in season, tides, and daylight cues, which act as "zeitgebers" that anchor the internal clock [1, 34].

2.1 Analytical methods

Analytical methods for identifying and quantifying circadian rhythmicity among a time series of data (e.g., 24 h HR recording) include *spectral analysis* or *least squares procedures* [34, 35]. While the *spectral analysis*, in particular, allows an easy access through visual inspection of an individual 24 h ECG recording (see also Section 4), the *least squares procedure* allows for group aggregation and statistical comparisons/analysis due to mathematical quantification of rhythmicity, as demonstrated in Section 3. Therefore, in an individual consultation setting, a summarizing graph is of particular value, while the latter allows for scientific comparisons to detect alterations in circadian parameters, e.g., in persons reporting a high vs. low number of depressive symptoms (see Section 3).

2.1.1 Spectral analysis

Using available commercial software, the 24 h measurement is first subdivided into separate intervals (5 minutes have become standard), and within these intervals, the frequency spectrum and the height of the amplitude (= energy density) are color-coded (see left panel of **Figure 1**; the spectral graphs were calculated using the commercial software Cardiscope™ ANALYTICS Professional Edition Version 1.2.156, HASIBA Medical GmbH, Austria). The array of each spectrum results in a colored two-dimensional image of the color-coded energy density. These images

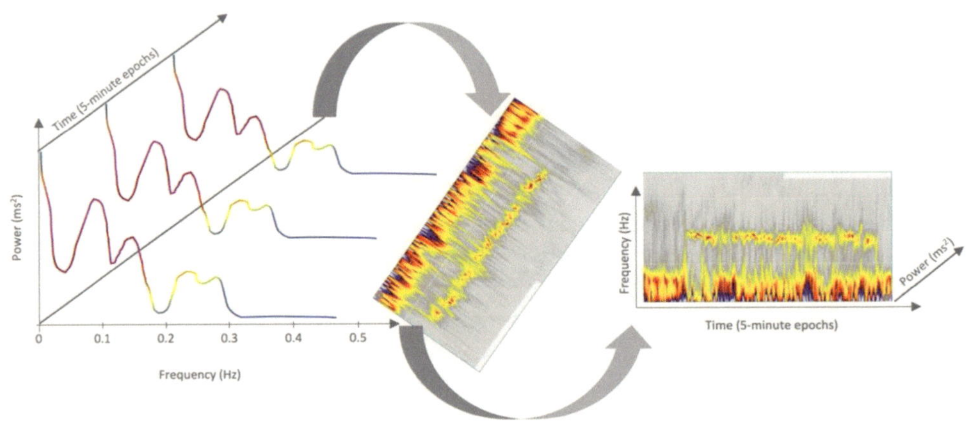

Figure 1.
Example of a color-coded power spectral segment (left panel) and its stacked representation of the 24 h time series (z-axis; right panel).

are stacked, introducing time as a third dimension, and of across frequency when viewed from a bird's eye perspective (see also **Figure 6**).

This individual graph, enhanced with diary information, can serve as a powerful tool in consultation (see Section 4).

2.1.2 Cosinor procedure

The cosinor procedure is suggested as the appropriate tool to detect circadian rhythmicity in cross-sectional studies with a single measurement [35]. In a first step, the 24 h recording is segmented into intervals, e.g., 5-minute intervals. In a 24 h recording, a total of 288 5-minute intervals are calculated. For each 5-minute interval, the HRV parameters need to be calculated.

Three individual-level cosine function parameters are estimated for each individual 24 h time series (now consisting of the 288 5-minute intervals) to quantify the circadian variation parameters of the selected HRV variables using the method of ordinary least squares regression (see Eq. (1)) [34]. Here, M is the midline-estimating statistic of rhythm (MESOR), a rhythm-adjusted mean, A is the amplitude (being the maximal distance between the oscillating signal and the MESOR), ϕ is the acrophase (defined as the clock time when A is reached), θ_i is the trigonometric angle, t_i is the sampling rate, P is the period (duration of one cycle, in this case, supposed to be 24 h), and e_i is the error term (**Figure 2**).

With the period P known, standard regression equations can be derived (see Eq. (2)) and analyzed using an ordinary least squares approach to minimize the residual sum of squared differences between observations and model estimation (see Eq. (3) and [34, 36, 37] for a comprehensive description).

$$Y_i = M + A\cos(\theta_i + \phi) + e_i \quad \text{where } \theta_i = \left(\frac{2\pi t_i}{P}\right) \tag{1}$$

$$\begin{aligned} Y_i &= M + \beta x + \gamma z + e_i \\ with&: \beta = A\cos\phi;\ \gamma = -A\sin\phi; \\ x &= \cos\left(\frac{2\pi t_i}{P}\right);\ z = \sin\left(\frac{2\pi t_i}{P}\right) \end{aligned} \tag{2}$$

$$RSS\ \Sigma_i \left[Y_i - \left(\hat{M} + \hat{\beta} x_i + \hat{\gamma} z_i\right)\right]^2 \tag{3}$$

Solving these equations provides the researcher with the three described variables per recording. In a second step, these can be easily used in further statistical analysis, as exemplified in the next section. Moreover, graphical between-group comparison including confidence intervals is possible (see examples in Section 3).

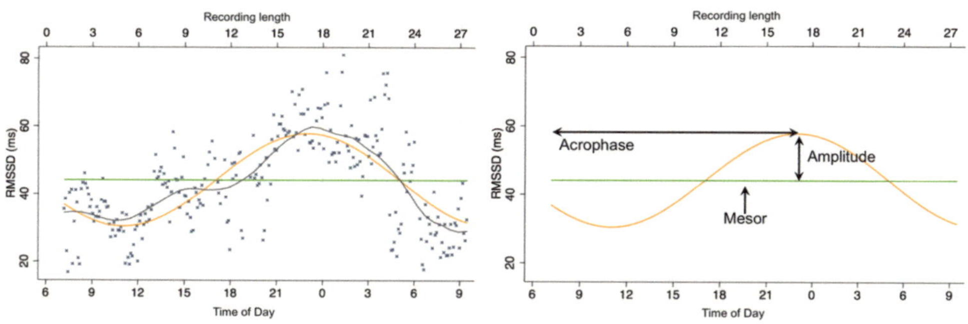

Figure 2.
Individual recording of 5-minute intervals of RMSSD (blue x on the left-hand panel) and the corresponding fitted cosine curve (orange) and LOWESS line (bluish-gray). The right-hand panel indicates the cosine measures that are calculated.

3. Examples of cosinor calculations detecting between-group differences of circadian HRV parameters

As with many other biomarkers, autonomic activity fluctuates in a pattern of diurnal variation with a frequency of an approximate solar day, with peak levels of vagal activity during nighttime in humans [21, 38, 39] and nonhuman primates [40]. Previous analyses by our group and other groups have demonstrated adverse or at least unfavorable intermediate health outcomes being associated with blunted circadian variation patterns, particularly with blunted or absent nighttime increase of vagal activity. This includes an elevated risk of cardiac events such as myocardial ischemia, myocardial infarction, malignant arrhythmias, and sudden cardiac death peaking in the early morning [41–44] as well as hyperglycemic states and elevated pro-inflammatory cytokines in a working population [21]. To use this information in daily work, a clinician needs reference values which are associated with clinical and preclinical conditions such as hyperglycemia. Only if these values exist, parameters can be used as a screening tool and help to identify individuals at risk in both clinical and nonclinical populations. In preventive settings, these parameters should be associated not only to somatic complaints but also to mental health conditions such as depressive symptoms. And finally, these parameters should index change, e.g., in a clinical population pre- to post-therapy or in occupational setting pre- to post-behavioral interventions.

Yet, reference values of circadian HRV parameter are scarce and of limited usefulness. For example, existing reference values of HRV (independent of diurnal variation) are based on varying recording length [45–49] with no reference to circadian variation, age, or sex. Studies reporting reference values based on 24 h recording length are analyzed with other time durations [50, 51] than the recommended 5-minute interval limiting comparability across studies or have a focus on young adults [52] or are based on rather small sample sizes (<200) [39, 52].

3.1 Reference values

We recently presented values for circadian variation of cardiac autonomic modulation in 931 rigorously healthy working adults (mean age 39 ± 10; 78% males) [31]. Consecutive 5-minute intervals of RMSSD were calculated from 24 h HR recordings that were collected at four distinct study sites of the Mannheim Industrial Cohort Study (MICS) in healthy working adults. "Healthy" was defined rigorously as indicating explicitly "no" to any of the following criteria (self-report): hypertension, dyslipidemia, hyperglycemia, respiratory diseases (e.g., asthma, COPD), angina pectoris, stroke, infarction, congenital heart defect (CHD), depression, burnout, other chronic diseases, cancer, and taking beta-blockers. First, three individual-level cosine function parameters were estimated to quantify the circadian variation as described in the previous section. Second, random-effect meta-analysis was used to estimate the impact of age group (18–24/25–34/35–44/55–65), shift work (Y/N), atypical employment (Y/N), the hierarchical position (division manager/project leader/employee/skilled worker/semiskilled worker), smoking, or being physically active on the three cosine parameters *MESOR*, *amplitude*, and ϕ. Results showed that older age and being female are associated with a significantly lower *amplitude*. Significant age decline in *MESOR* could be observed. Particularly, age-related decline in *MESOR* and *amplitude* was more pronounced in the younger age groups (see **Figure 3**). In addition, two age groups showed phase advances compared to the youngest age group. Interestingly, current smoking was associated with reduced *MESOR*, while physical activity was associated with increased *MESOR*. Working any kind of shift work is associated

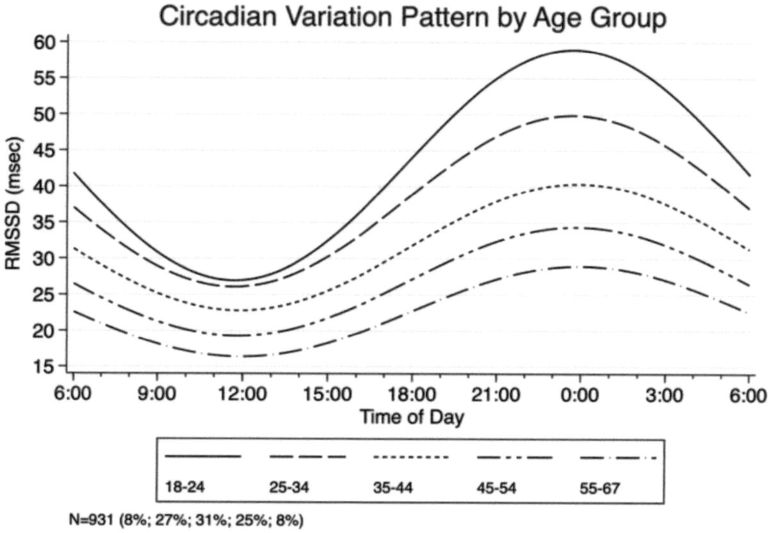

Figure 3.
Circadian variation pattern of RMSSD by age from N=931 rigorously healthy working adults of the MICS-cohort.

with higher oscillation in *amplitude*. Particularly, age declined in both the overall mean (= *MESOR*) and the oscillation (*amplitude*) indicating a decrease of nocturnal parasympathetic activity.

3.2 Test-retest reliability of circadian variation patterns

To the best of our knowledge, no study has yet investigated the short- or long-term reproducibility of circadian variation patterns of HRV parameters. We recently demonstrated short-term reliability in 74 men (age 41 ± 7) with repeated 24 h measures and a gap of 1 day between measures [53]. The vagal activity was indicated using estimates of HRV (RMSSD, pNN50, SDNN). Between-day associations were calculated using Pearson's correlation (PC). Short-term reliability was assessed using intra-class correlation (ICC) and Bland-Altman analysis (bias ± limits of agreement). The results demonstrate an excellent ICC (all > 0.82) and PC (all > 0.83) for the *MESOR*. *Amplitude* measures were good (ICC and PC > 0.71) for RMSSD and pNN50 but fair (ICC and PC < 0.60) for SDNN. Acrophase measures were fair (ICC and PC all < 0.60). Bland-Altman plots showed no systematic bias between measurement days for any measure. This study demonstrates high reliability for the rhythm-adjusted 24 h mean in primarily vagally mediated and mixed measures in men. As hypothesized, lower but still good reliability was demonstrated for the *amplitude* in vagally mediated HRV measures. This indicates a higher day-to-day variability of the vagally mediated HRV amplitude parameters and more trait-like *MESOR* parameters. However, future studies need to expand to female samples, collect potential (time lagged) determinates of the diurnal variation using ecological momentary assessments, and investigate the long-term test-retest reliability.

3.3 Depressive symptoms and circadian variation patterns

We also demonstrated previously a salient association between circadian variation patterns and depressive symptoms in 3030 predominantly healthy employees (mean age 41 ± 7; females 20.2%) [54]. Multivariate linear regression models revealed a negative association with *MESOR* and *amplitude* in men, but the

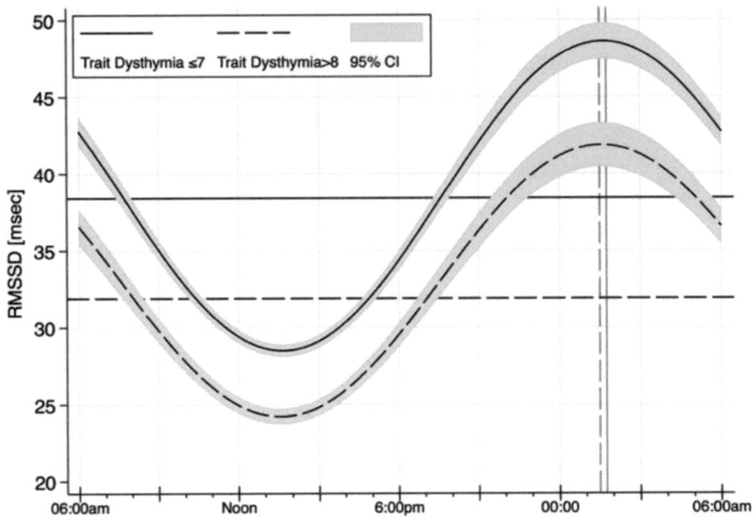

Figure 4.
Patterns of circadian rhythms of vagal activity vary by trait measures of dysthymia.

opposite in women. This pattern of findings indicates an important moderation effect of sex in the association of circadian variation patterns with RMSSD and depressive symptoms in a healthy (preclinical) population. These findings were partly replicated by investigating associations between affective trait measures with circadian variation patterns of RMSSD [55]. Here, trait measures of positive and negative affect in N = 81 male employees (mean age 41 ± 7) were significantly associated with *MESOR* in multivariate linear regression models. **Figure 4** exemplifies the results by showing the predicted diurnal variation of RMSSD by a median split of the negative affect scale and its corresponding *MESOR* line and θ around 1:30 a.m. It still needs to be explored if the decrement of circadian variation can be (partly) reversed if symptoms decrease. Two randomized controlled trials currently investigate the changes of circadian variation patterns of HRV pre- to post-therapy (DRKS00016616; NCT03080025).

3.4 Inflammatory markers and circadian variation patterns

The inflammatory reflex is a physiological mechanism through which the vagus nerve regulates immune function [56]. Here, efferent vagal activity inhibits the release of pro-inflammatory cytokines via the release of acetylcholine and has been termed the cholinergic anti-inflammatory pathway [57–59]. Moreover, the release of interleukin-6 (IL-6) and other cytokines triggers the hepatic synthesis of C-reactive protein (CRP) [60]. In addition, the vagus nerve is also known to relay information about the peripheral immune status to the brain via IL-1 receptors conveyed by paraganglia cells situated in parasympathetic ganglia [61]. Thus, both vagal efferent and afferent pathways seem to play an important role in immune regulation. We previously demonstrated that decreased vagally mediated HRV at baseline predicted increased low-grade systemic inflammation (a marker of CHD risk) after 4 years in healthy working adults [19]. The circadian variation pattern of RMSSD shows an association with systemic low-grade inflammation [62]. Data were collected at four distinct study sites of the Mannheim Industrial Cohort Study (MICS) in 3134 healthy working adults (mean age 42 ± 11; 80% males). Low-grade inflammation was measured by high-sensitive C-reactive protein (hsCRP).

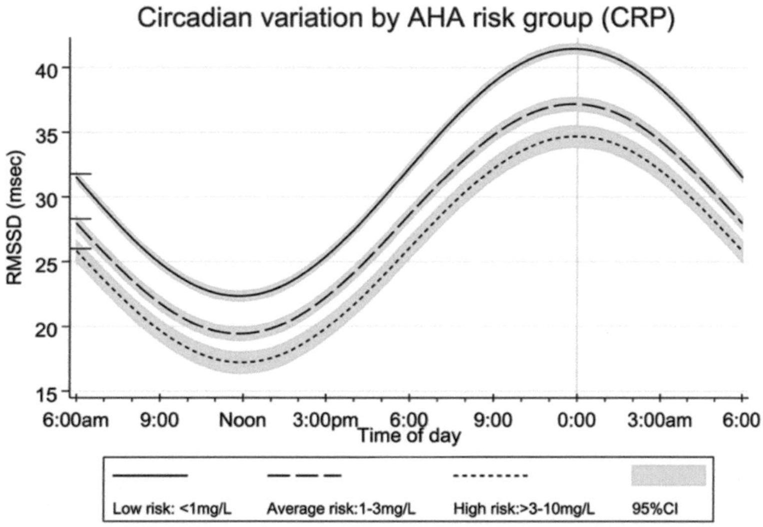

Figure 5.
Circadian variation in groups with different systemic inflammation levels as defined by the American Heart Association (AHA).

Participants with acute inflammation (hsCRP >10 mg/L) were excluded. CRP was categorized into the risk groups defined by the American Heart Association (AHA) as follows: low-risk group (<1 mg/L), medium-risk group (1–3 mg/L), and high-risk group (>3 mg/L). In the present study, lower *MESOR* and higher *amplitude* were associated with elevated levels of low-grade inflammation (see **Figure 5**).

4. Examples of 24 h HRV patterns in practical application

4.1 Clinical population

As described in the introduction, reduced HRV parameters have been shown in different risk states and diseases including depression [63]. At the same time, disturbances of circadian rhythms have been described in depression [64]. A 24 h measurement of HRV can help to detect the degree of disturbance that has already occurred. Furthermore, it supports recovery by identifying resources that can be enhanced and strengthened. Recovery from a chronobiologic point of view includes not only reduction in, e.g., depressive symptoms, but also restoration of chronobiologic rhythms. Repeated measurements can document the process of recovery and the effect of interventions.

Considering these points, a 24 h measurement of HRV could prove itself as a helpful psychophysiological tool in a psychotherapeutic setting. However, to the best of our knowledge, 24 h HRV was not yet implemented in this kind of setting. Therefore, we designed a study implementing 24 h HRV measurements into a psychosomatic consultation at the workplace (trial-ID German Clinical Trials Register DRKS00012473). The psychosomatic consultation at the workplace is a service of the Department of Psychosomatic Medicine and Psychotherapy at Ulm University Medical Center (Germany) and has been described in detail elsewhere [65]. In brief, it is open to employees who receive an early consultation by a doctor or a psychologist specialized in psychotherapy for all personnel reporting psychic (e.g., depressive symptoms, anxiety) and potentially psychosomatic complaints such as

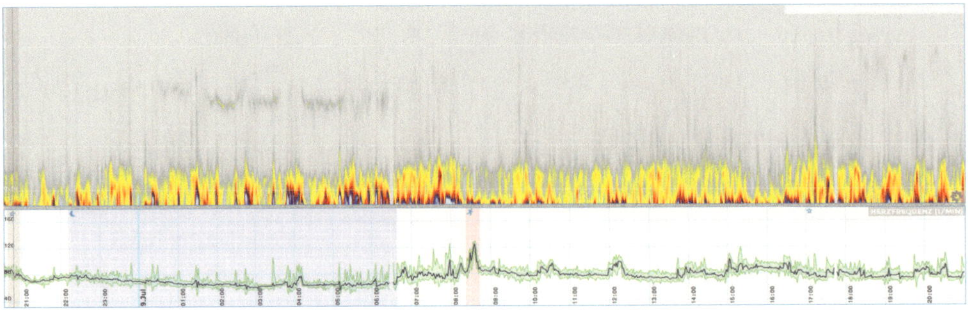

Figure 6.
24 h HRV measurement of a patient with major depression. Displayed are heart rate and spectral analyses.

back pain, sleep problems, and exhaustion. It comprises two parts—the diagnostic phase (max. three sessions) and the immediate short-term intervention of another max. 9 sessions (if indicated). The study took place at a large center for disabled care in Germany. HRV was measured after the first sessions and the results were discussed with the patients in the second or third session. All patients that continued the sessions received a second 24 h HRV measurement at the end of the intervention (marker of change). The study also covered disturbances of the hypothalamic pituitary adrenal (HPA) axis by collecting eight saliva samples for a cortisol day profile.

Recruitment was completed in May 2019, but repeated measurements are still ongoing, so final statistical analyses will be reported later. Preliminary findings suggest that about 50% of the patients were willing to participate in the study and that all patients that were offered a second measurement (i.e., all patients receiving a short-term intervention) completed the second measurement. The vast majority of patients indicated that they gained new insights in psychophysiological interactions and most of them (90%) would highly recommend the consultation (particularly the HRV measurement with feedback) to a close friend.

Here, we want to present a case with a major depressive episode. A 50-year-old man presented with depressed mood, diminished interest in all activities, fatigue, problems to concentrate at work, and sleeping disturbances with problems falling asleep, waking up in the middle of the night and in the morning, and lying awake for a longer time. He also complained about restlessness which had become better by starting medication with olanzapine 2.5 mg per day. Twenty-four hour HRV analyses revealed a pronounced overall reduction in variability as well as a reduced night-day variation (see **Figure 6**). At night, vagal indices normally increase. In this patient, RMSSD and HF power were low throughout the day and the night, confirming his subjective complaints of unrestful sleep (**Table 1**). His chronobiologic rhythms are obviously disrupted to a greater extent on the basis of an overall reduction in variability that does not allow much variation throughout the day. Searching for resources led to one single time point at about 5 o'clock in the afternoon where power spectral analyses show for a short time signals in the VLF, LF, and HF power band. The patient reported that at this time, he sat down in his garden and could enjoy the air and the birds singing for a while.

The symptoms aggravated in the following 2 weeks so that he was transferred to a hospital with psychiatric inpatient care.

4.2 Preventive setting

As discussed in the introduction, 24 h measurement of HRV may be a practical tool in preventive settings like occupational health. We implemented it in three large enterprises of the industrial, automotive, and metal sector into a regular

Parameter	Unit	Total	Daytime	Sleep
Duration	hh:mm	24:30	16:02	08:26
Mean HR	/min	75	80	67
SDNN	ms	99.5	72,6	76.9
rMSSD	ms	15.2	14,6	16.4
Total power-i	ms^2	1643	1461	1991
VLF-i	ms^2	1082	888	1454
LF-i	ms^2	407	417	387
HF-i	ms^2	70	66	79

Abbreviations: HR, heart rate; SDNN, standard deviation of normal interbeat intervals; RMSSD, root mean square of successive differences; VLF, very low frequency; LF, low frequency; HF, high frequency.
-i indicates that this value is calculated as a mean of the values of all 5-min timeframes.

Table 1.
HRV indices of a patient with major depression.

manager health checkup and as an offer for any manager and employee who presents at the occupational health physician (trial-ID German Clinical Trials Register DRKS00014653). First, we want to show a healthy example with intact chronobiology and after that an example out of the mentioned study with clear disturbances.

The first example shows the measurement results of a 36-year-old woman. The medical history contained no diagnoses, no medication, normal weight, and normal blood pressure. She was working part time, about 30 h/week, living with her husband and with three children. Alcohol consumption was moderate, and she engaged in sports activities of 3–4 h/week. She complaint feeling tired in the morning and sometimes during the day but reported falling asleep easily in the evening and sleeping well. Scores for irritation and depression showed low values, while the stress scale showed intermediate values, where she was reporting work piling up.

HRV analyses showed a pronounced and instant decrease of heart rate at night, with a distinct increase in RMSSD and HF. In spectral analyses, the nighttime is easily detected by a specific pattern inside the HF power band which represents respiratory sinus arrhythmia (RSA). In this healthy example, RSA is present almost throughout the whole night, with changing patterns in the LF power band as it is typical for sleep cycles. This is an example of well-functioning chronobiology. The daytime also shows variability with different patterns, e.g., at lunch break around 12 o'clock, during sports activity around 3 o'clock in the afternoon, and in the evening at home (see **Figure 7** and **Table 2**).

The second example shows the results of a measurement a 50-year-old male manager working full time about 40 h/week. He also had no diagnosed diseases and reported no medication. Weight and blood pressure were unobtrusive. He reported a moderate alcohol consumption and moderate sports activity of 1–2 h/week. His complaints were only some back pain from time to time. He reported almost half of the nights waking up in the middle of the night with problems continuing sleeping and marked his sleep as "fair." Irritation scale was low with only sometimes being irritated. No depressive or anxious symptoms were present.

In the spectral analyses (**Figure 8**), the typical RSA pattern at night is missing. Generally, the power seems to be "cut" with almost no spikes entering the HF power band. Though heart rate decreased at night, all HRV parameters, especially vagal values, were reduced at night, which is an inverted state. HR decreased only slowly and reached the lowest values after 4 o'clock and 5 h of sleep, respectively. Analyses of his daytime activity showed no breaks throughout the whole day and 1 h of a vigorous sports activity (ball game) from 20 to 21 o'clock with a mean HR of 130/min and a max

HR of 170/min (**Table 3**). Heart rate did not return to baseline for 2 h, which indicates overtraining. The first hours of sleep show reduced variability in all power bands, a pattern that stands for exhaustion. Allover, chronobiologic rhythms are markedly disturbed, though HRV indices are still higher than in the example with major depression.

The consultation revealed a highly ambitious personality who was used to well-functioning of his body all of the time and who a mostly postpones the needs of his body in order to solve a problem on the job or to win the game at sports. The graph helped to intriguingly demonstrate to the manager the impact of what he is doing to his body and motivated him to learn to perceive when he reaches his limits as well as to hold on to his limit and not try to overachieve.

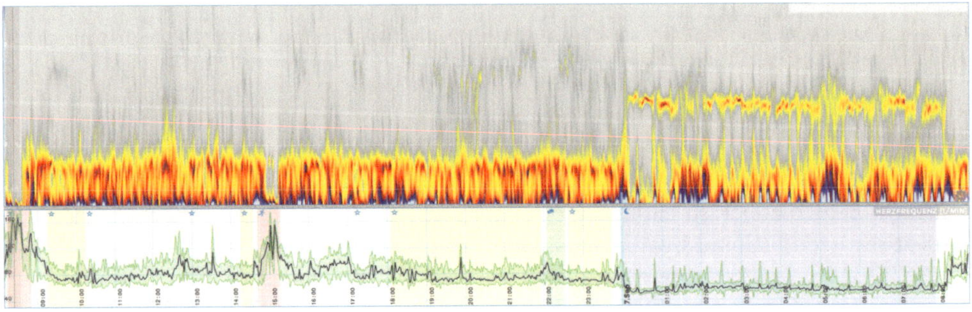

Figure 7.
24 h HRV measurement of a healthy, 36-year-old woman. Displayed are heart rate and spectral analyses.

Parameter	Unit	Total	Daytime	Sleep
Duration	hh:mm	24:41	16:44	07:57
Mean HR	/min	74	83	55
SDNN	ms	206.2	144.6	104.7
rMSSD	ms	34.8	30.3	46.0
Total power-i	ms^2	5305	4794	6364
VLF-i	ms^2	3105	2596	4160
LF-i	ms^2	1525	1650	1266
HF-i	ms^2	412	281	684

Abbreviations: HR, heart rate; SDNN, standard deviation of normal interbeat intervals; RMSSD, root mean square of successive differences; VLF, very low frequency; LF, low frequency; HF, high frequency.
-i indicates that this value is calculated as a mean of the values of all 5-min timeframes.

Table 2.
HRV indices of a healthy, 36-year-old woman.

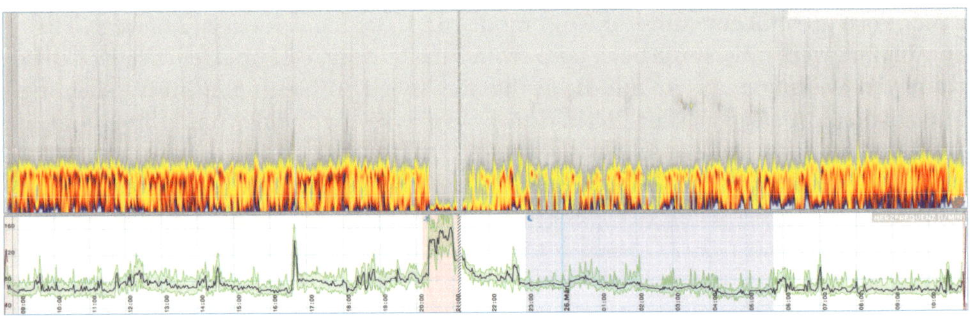

Figure 8.
24 h HRV measurement of a 50-year-old manager. Displayed are heart rate and spectral analyses.

Parameter	Unit	Total	Day	Sleep
Duration	hh:mm	26:27	19:44	6:43
Mean HR	/min	74	76	69
SDNN	ms	148.0	155.1	98.0
rMSSD	ms	21.4	22.7	16.5
Total power-i	ms^2	3630	3980	2657
VLF-i	ms^2	2086	2221	1714
LF-i	ms^2	1248	1410	800
HF-i	ms^2	82	95	46

Abbreviations: HR, heart rate; SDNN, standard deviation of normal interbeat intervals; RMSSD, root mean square of successive differences; VLF, very low frequency; LF, low frequency; HF, high frequency.
-i indicates that this value is calculated as a mean of the values of all 5-min timeframes.

Table 3.
HRV indices of a 50-year-old manager.

5. Conclusion

HRV as a chronobiologic, disease-unspecific biomarker holds the possibility to become a screening tool in preventive settings as well as a tool to monitor overall health status, e.g., pre- to post-therapy, and serve as an instrument to demonstrate to a patient the physiological reactions to his specific environmental cues. This could be beneficial to persons usually not so open to talk about feelings and thus pave the way into a conversation about psychosomatic interactions. Thus, its psychophysiological nature mirroring somatic as well as mental states implies HRV as a well-suited psychosomatic marker. Its usefulness in these settings should be further explored.

Acknowledgements

Parts of this work were conducted at the Leadership Personality Center in Ulm (Germany) with the support of the Karl Schlecht foundation.

MNJ positions were funded between 2016 and 2017 through the physician scientist program (Medical Faculty Heidelberg, Heidelberg University, Germany). The other studies were funded through internal funds of the Mannheim Institute of Public Health, Social and Preventive Medicine (Heidelberg University), the Institute for Medical Psychology (Center for Psychosocial Medicine, Heidelberg University), and the Clinic for Psychosomatic Medicine and Psychotherapy (University Medical Center Ulm).

JJM is awarded with a funding from the Canadian Institutes of Health Research and Fonds de Recherche du Québec-Santé that supports this work.

None of the funding entities had a role in data analysis, result report, or interpretation of this work.

Conflict of interest

EMB, MNJ and JJM declare to have no conflict of interest.

Author details

Marc N. Jarczok[1*], Harald Guendel[1], Jennifer J. McGrath[2] and Elisabeth M. Balint[3,1]

1 Department of Psychosomatic Medicine and Psychotherapy, Ulm University Medical Center, Ulm, Germany

2 PERFORM Centre, Montreal, Quebec, Canada

3 Leadership Personality Center Ulm (LPCU), Ulm University, Ulm, Germany

*Address all correspondence to: marc.jarczok@gmail.com

References

[1] Astiz M, Heyde I, Oster H. Mechanisms of communication in the mammalian circadian timing system. International Journal of Molecular Sciences. 2019;**20**(2)

[2] Singh RB, Cornélissen G, Weydahl A, Schwartzkopff O, Katinas G, Otsuka K, et al. Circadian heart rate and blood pressure variability considered for research and patient care. International Journal of Cardiology. 2003;**87**(1):9-28; discussion 29-30. Available from: http://www.ncbi.nlm.nih.gov/pubmed/12468050

[3] Halberg F, Cornélissen G, Wall D, Otsuka K, Halberg J, Katinas G, et al. Engineering and governmental challenge: 7-day/24-hour chronobiologic blood pressure and heart rate screening: Part I. Biomedical Instrumentation & Technology. 2003;**36**(2):89-122. Available from: http://www.ncbi.nlm.nih.gov/pubmed/11938620

[4] Report IAG. Gefährdungsbeurteilung psychischer Belastungen—Tipps zum Einstieg. 2013

[5] Stalder T, Kirschbaum C, Kudielka BM, Adam EK, Pruessner JC, Wüst S, et al. Assessment of the cortisol awakening response: Expert consensus guidelines. Psychoneuroendocrinology. 2016;**63**:414-432. Available from: http://www.ncbi.nlm.nih.gov/pubmed/26563991

[6] Mauss D, Jarczok MN, Fischer JE. A streamlined approach for assessing the Allostatic Load Index in industrial employees. Stress. 2015;**18**(4):475-483. Available from: http://informahealthcare.com/doi/abs/10.3109/10253890.2015.1040987

[7] Mauss D, Li J, Schmidt B, Angerer P, Jarczok MN. Measuring allostatic load in the workforce: A systematic review. Industrial Health. 2015;**53**(1):5-20. Available from: https://www.jstage.jst.go.jp/article/indhealth/53/1/53_2014-0122/_article

[8] Mauss D, Jarczok MN, Fischer JE. The streamlined Allostatic Load Index: A replication of study results. Stress. 2016;**3890**(August):1-20. Available from: http://www.tandfonline.com/doi/full/10.1080/10253890.2016.1219718

[9] Stephens C, Alpass F, Towers A, Stevenson B. The effects of types of social networks, perceived social support, and loneliness on the health of older people: Accounting for the social context. Journal of Aging and Health. 2011;**23**(6):887-911

[10] Seeman TE, Singer BH, Rowe JW, Horwitz RI, McEwen BS. Price of adaptation—Allostatic load and its health consequences. MacArthur studies of successful aging. Archives of Internal Medicine. 1997;**157**(19):2259-2268. Available from: http://www.ncbi.nlm.nih.gov/pubmed/9343003

[11] McEwen B, Nasveld P, Palmer M, Anderson R. Allostatic Load—A Review of the Literature. Canberra: Department of Veterans' Affairs; 2012

[12] Wulsin L, Herman J, Thayer JF. Stress, autonomic imbalance, and the prediction of metabolic risk: A model and a proposal for research. Neuroscience & Biobehavioral Reviews. 2018;**86**(December):12-20. Available from: http://linkinghub.elsevier.com/retrieve/pii/S0149763417304529

[13] Thayer JF, Lane RD. A model of neurovisceral integration in emotion regulation and dysregulation. Journal of Affective Disorders. 2000;**61**(3):201-216. Available from: http://www.ncbi.nlm.nih.gov/pubmed/11163422

[14] Bernard C. Lecture on the physiology of the heart and its connections with

the brain, delivered at the Sorbonne, the 27th March, 1865. Tr. by J. S. Morel. 1st ed. Savannah: Purse & Son.; 1867. Available from: 39002086349314.med.yale.edu

[15] Shaffer F, Ginsberg JP. An overview of heart rate variability metrics and norms. Frontiers in Public Health, September. 2017;**5**:258. Available from: http://journal.frontiersin.org/article/10.3389/fpubh.2017.00258/full

[16] Thayer JF, Ahs F, Fredrikson M, Sollers JJ, Wager TD. A meta-analysis of heart rate variability and neuroimaging studies: Implications for heart rate variability as a marker of stress and health. Neuroscience and Biobehavioral Reviews. 2012;**36**(2):747-756. Available from: http://www.ncbi.nlm.nih.gov/pubmed/22178086

[17] Kemp AH, Koenig J, Thayer JF. From psychological moments to mortality: A multidisciplinary synthesis on heart rate variability spanning the continuum of time. Neuroscience & Biobehavioral Reviews. 2017;**83**(March):547-567. DOI: 10.1016/j.neubiorev.2017.09.006

[18] Aeschbacher S, Schoen T, Dörig L, Kreuzmann R, Neuhauser C, Schmidt-Trucksäss A, et al. Heart rate, heart rate variability and inflammatory biomarkers among young and healthy adults. Annals of Medicine. 2017;**49**(1):32-41

[19] Jarczok MN, Koenig J, Mauss D, Fischer JE, Thayer JF. Lower heart rate variability predicts increased level of C-reactive protein 4 years later in healthy, nonsmoking adults. Journal of Internal Medicine. 2014;**276**:667-671. Available from: http://doi.wiley.com/10.1111/joim.12295

[20] Thayer JF, Fischer JE. Heart rate variability, overnight urinary norepinephrine and C-reactive protein: Evidence for the cholinergic anti-inflammatory pathway in healthy human adults. Journal of Internal Medicine. 2009;**265**(4):439-447. Available from: http://www.ncbi.nlm.nih.gov/pubmed/19019182

[21] Jarczok LJ, Mauss D, Fischer JE, Thayer JF. Heart rate variability is associated with glycemic status after controlling for components of the metabolic syndrome. International Journal of Cardiology. 2013;**167**(3):855-861. Available from: http://linkinghub.elsevier.com/retrieve/pii/S0167527312001398

[22] Thayer JF, Lane RD. The role of vagal function in the risk for cardiovascular disease and mortality. Biological Psychology. 2007;**74**(2):224-242

[23] Fagundes CP, Murray DM, Hwang BS, Gouin J-P, Thayer JF, Sollers JJ, et al. Sympathetic and parasympathetic activity in cancer-related fatigue: More evidence for a physiological substrate in cancer survivors. Psychoneuroendocrinology. 2011;**36**(8):1137-1147. Available from: http://www.pubmedcentral.nih.gov/articlerender.fcgi?artid=3128662&tool=pmcentrez&rendertype=abstract

[24] Loerbroks A, Schilling O, Haxsen V, Jarczok MN, Thayer JF, Fischer JE. The fruits of ones labor: Effort-reward imbalance but not job strain is related to heart rate variability across the day in 35-44-year-old workers. Journal of Psychosomatic Research. 2010;**69**(2):151-159. Available from: http://linkinghub.elsevier.com/retrieve/pii/S0022399910001169?showall=true

[25] Koenig J, Jarczok MN, Ellis RJ, Hillecke TK, Thayer JF. Heart rate variability and experimentally induced pain in healthy adults: A systematic review. European Journal of Pain. 2013;**18**(3):301-314. Available from: http://www.ncbi.nlm.nih.gov/pubmed/23922336

[26] Henderson LA, Gandevia SC, Macefield VG. Somatotopic

organization of the processing of muscle and cutaneous pain in the left and right insula cortex: A single-trial fMRI study. Pain. 2007;**128**(1-2):20-30. Available from: http://www.ncbi.nlm.nih.gov/pubmed/17011704

[27] Weiss T, Straube T, Boettcher J, Hecht H, Spohn D, Miltner WHR. Brain activation upon selective stimulation of cutaneous C- and Adelta-fibers. NeuroImage. 2008;**41**(4):1372-1381. Available from: http://www.ncbi.nlm.nih.gov/pubmed/18499480

[28] Pereira EAC, Green AL, Bradley KM, Soper N, Moir L, Stein JF, et al. Regional cerebral perfusion differences between periventricular grey, thalamic and dual target deep brain stimulation for chronic neuropathic pain. Stereotactic and Functional Neurosurgery. 2007;**85**(4):175-183. Available from: http://www.ncbi.nlm.nih.gov/pubmed/17389817

[29] Kemp AH, Brunoni AR, Santos IS, Nunes MA, Dantas EM, Carvalho de Figueiredo R, et al. Effects of depression, anxiety, comorbidity, and antidepressants on resting-state heart rate and its variability: An ELSA-Brasil cohort baseline study. The American Journal of Psychiatry. 2014;**171**(12):1328-1334

[30] Jarczok MN, Kleber ME, Koenig J, Loerbroks A, Herr RM, Hoffmann K, et al. Investigating the mechanisms of self-rated health: Heart rate variability is more strongly associated than other frequently used biomarkers in a cross sectional occupational sample. PLoS One. 2015:1-19. DOI: 10.1371/journal.pone.0117196

[31] Jarczok MN, Koenig J, Fischer JE, Hoffmann K, Schmidt B, Mauss D, et al. Circadian variation of cardiac autonomic modulation in a rigorously healthy working population: Results from the MICS-Cohort. Psychosomatic Medicine. 2015;**77**(3)

[32] Garakani A, Martinez JM, Aaronson CJ, Voustianiouk A, Kaufmann H, Gorman JM. Effect of medication and psychotherapy on heart rate variability in panic disorder. Depression and Anxiety. 2009;**26**(3):251-258

[33] Deboer T. Sleep homeostasis and the circadian clock: Do the circadian pacemaker and the sleep homeostat influence each other's functioning? Neurobiology of Sleep and Circadian Rhythms. 2018;**5**(March):68-77. DOI: 10.1016/j.nbscr.2018.02.003

[34] Cornelissen G. Cosinor-based rhythmometry. Theoretical Biology and Medical Modelling. 2014;**11**(1):16. Available from: http://www.tbiomed.com/content/11/1/16

[35] Refinetti R, Cornélissen G, Halberg F. Procedures for numerical analysis of circadian rhythms. Biological Rhythm Research. 2007;**38**(4):275-325. Available from: http://www.pubmedcentral.nih.gov/articlerender.fcgi?artid=3663600&tool=pmcentrez&rendertype=abstract

[36] Fernández JR, Hermida RC, Mojón A. Chronobiological analysis techniques. Application to blood pressure. Philosophical Transactions. Series A, Mathematical, Physical, and Engineering Sciences. 2009;**367**(1887):431-445. Available from: http://www.ncbi.nlm.nih.gov/pubmed/18940774

[37] Minors DS, Waterhouse JM. Mathematical and statistical analysis of circadian rhythms. Psychoneuroendocrinology. 1988;**13**(6):443-464

[38] Huikuri HV, Niemelä MJ, Ojala S, Rantala A, Ikäheimo MJ, Airaksinen KE. Circadian rhythms of frequency domain measures of heart rate variability in healthy subjects and patients with coronary artery disease.

Effects of arousal and upright posture. Circulation. 1994;**90**(1):121-126. Available from: http://www.ncbi.nlm.nih.gov/pubmed/8025987

[39] Li X, Shaffer ML, Rodriguez-Colon S, He F, Wolbrette DL, Alagona P, et al. The circadian pattern of cardiac autonomic modulation in a middle-aged population. Clinical Autonomic Research. 2011;**21**(3):143-150. Available from: http://www.pubmedcentral.nih.gov/articlerender.fcgi?artid=3093547&tool=pmcentrez&rendertype=abstract

[40] Jarczok MN, Koenig J, Shively CA, Thayer JF. Behavioral depression is associated with increased vagally mediated heart rate variability in adult female cynomolgus monkeys (*Macaca fascicularis*). International Journal of Psychophysiology. 2018;**131**:139-143. Available from: http://linkinghub.elsevier.com/retrieve/pii/S0167876017302507

[41] Bernardi L, Ricordi L, Lazzari P, Soldá P, Calciati A, Ferrari MR, et al. Impaired circadian modulation of sympathovagal activity in diabetes. A possible explanation for altered temporal onset of cardiovascular disease. Circulation. 1992;**86**(5):1443-1452. Available from: http://www.ncbi.nlm.nih.gov/pubmed/1423958

[42] Carney RM, Steinmeyer B, Freedland KE, Stein PK, Hayano J, Blumenthal JA, et al. Nocturnal patterns of heart rate and the risk of mortality after acute myocardial infarction. American Heart Journal. 2014;**168**(1):117-125. Available from: http://www.ncbi.nlm.nih.gov/pubmed/24952868

[43] Huikuri HV, Linnaluoto MK, Seppänen T, Airaksinen KEJ, Kessler KM, Takkunen JT, et al. Circadian rhythm of heart rate variability in survivors of cardiac arrest. The American Journal of Cardiology. 1992;**70**(6):610-615. Available from: http://www.ncbi.nlm.nih.gov/pubmed/1510009

[44] Muller JE, Tofler GH, Stone PH. Circadian variation and triggers of onset of acute cardiovascular disease. Circulation. 1989;**79**(4):733-743. Available from: http://circ.ahajournals.org/cgi/doi/10.1161/01.CIR.79.4.733

[45] Koenig J, Jarczok MN, Warth M, Ellis RJ, Bach C, Hillecke TK, et al. Body mass index is related to autonomic nervous system activity as measured by heart rate variability—A replication using short term measurements. Journal of Nutrition, Health and Aging. 2014;**18**(3):300-302. Available from: http://www.ncbi.nlm.nih.gov/pubmed/24626758

[46] Seppälä S, Laitinen T, Tarvainen MP, Tompuri T, Veijalainen A, Savonen K, et al. Normal values for heart rate variability parameters in children 6-8 years of age: The PANIC Study. Clinical Physiology and Functional Imaging. 2014;**34**(4):290-296

[47] Liao D, Crow RS, Folsom AR, Swenne CA, Schouten EG, Hannan PJ, et al. Low heart rate variability in a 2-minute rhythm strip predicts risk of coronary heart disease and mortality from several causes: The ARIC study. Atherosclerosis risk in communities. Circulation. 2000;**102**(11):1239-1244

[48] Baek HJ, Cho C-H, Cho J, Woo J-M. Reliability of ultra-short-term analysis as a surrogate of standard 5-min analysis of heart rate variability. Telemedicine Journal and E-Health. 2015;**21**(5):404-414. Available from: http://www.ncbi.nlm.nih.gov/pubmed/25807067

[49] Jarrin DC, McGrath JJ, Poirier P, Séguin L, Tremblay RE, Montplaisir JY, et al. Short-term heart rate variability in a population-based sample of 10-year-old children. Pediatric Cardiology. 2015;**36**(1):41-48

[50] Bonnemeier H, Richardt G, Potratz J, Wiegand UKH, Brandes A, Kluge N, et al. Circadian profile of cardiac autonomic nervous modulation in healthy subjects: Differing effects of aging and gender on heart rate variability. Journal of Cardiovascular Electrophysiology. 2003;**14**(8):791-799. Available from: http://www.ncbi.nlm.nih.gov/pubmed/12890036

[51] Umetani K, Duda CL, Singer DH. Aging effects on cycle length dependence of heart rate variability. In: Biomedical Engineering Conference 1996. Dayton, OH, USA: IEEE; 1996. pp. 361-364

[52] Nakagawa M, Iwao T, Ishida S, Yonemochi H, Fujino T, Saikawa T, et al. Circadian rhythm of the signal averaged electrocardiogram and its relation to heart rate variability in healthy subjects. Heart. 1998;**79**(5):493-496 Available from: http://www.ncbi.nlm.nih.gov/pubmed/9659198

[53] Jarczok MN, Koenig J, Aguilar-Raab C, Diepolder M-L, Traunmueller C, Thayer JF, et al. Test-retest reliability of parameters indexing circadian variation in vagal activity. Psychosomatic Medicine. 2017;**79**(4):A42

[54] Jarczok MN, Aguilar-Raab C, Koenig J, Kaess M, Borniger JC, Nelson RJ, et al. The Heart's rhythm "n" blues: Sex differences in circadian variation patterns of vagal activity vary by depressive symptoms in predominantly healthy employees. Chronobiology International. 2018;**0528**:1-14. Available from: https://www.tandfonline.com/doi/full/10.1080/07420528.2018.1439499

[55] Jarczok MN, Warth M, Gabel C, Koenig J, Aguilar-Raab C, Traunmuller C, et al. Patterns of circadian rhythms of vagal activity vary by trait measures of euthymia and dysthymia. Psychosomatic Medicine. 2017;**79**(4):A6

[56] Pavlov VA, Tracey KJ. Neural regulation of immunity: Molecular mechanisms and clinical translation. Nature Neuroscience. 2017;**20**(2): 156-166. Available from: http://www.ncbi.nlm.nih.gov/pubmed/28092663

[57] Tracey KJ. Understanding immunity requires more than immunology. Nature Immunology. 2010;**11**(7):561-564. Available from: http://www.ncbi.nlm.nih.gov/pubmed/20562838

[58] Matteoli G, Boeckxstaens GE. The vagal innervation of the gut and immune homeostasis. Gut. 2013;**62**(8):1214-1222. Available from: http://www.pubmedcentral.nih.gov/articlerender.fcgi?artid=3711371&tool=pmcentrez&rendertype=abstract

[59] VA P, Tracey KJ. The vagus nerve and the inflammatory reflex—Linking immunity and metabolism. Nature Reviews. Endocrinology. 2012;**8**(12):743-754. Available from: http://www.ncbi.nlm.nih.gov/pubmed/23169440

[60] Casas JP, Shah T, Hingorani a D, Danesh J, Pepys MB. C-reactive protein and coronary heart disease: A critical review. Journal of Internal Medicine. 2008;**264**(4):295-314. Available from: http://www.ncbi.nlm.nih.gov/pubmed/18823504

[61] Sternberg EM. Neural regulation of innate immunity: A coordinated nonspecific host response to pathogens. Nature Reviews Immunology. 2006;**6**(4):318-328. Available from: http://www.pubmedcentral.nih.gov/articlerender.fcgi?artid=1783839&tool=pmcentrez&rendertype=abstract

[62] Jarczok MN, Koenig J, Bosch JA, Fischer JE, Thayer JF. Circadian variation of cardiac autonomic modulation and low-grade inflammation in working adults. Psychosomatic Medicine. 2017;**77**(3). Available from:

http://content.wkhealth.com/linkback/openurl?sid=WKPTLP:landingpage&an=00006842-201504000-00018

[63] Kemp AH. Major depressive disorder with melancholia displays robust alterations in resting state heart rate and its variability: Implications for future morbidity and mortality. Frontiers in Psychology, November. 2014;**5**:1-9

[64] Germain A, Kupfer DJ. Circadian rhythm disturbances in depression. Human Psychopharmacology. 2008;**23**(7):571-585

[65] Rothermund E, Kilian R, Hoelzer M, Rieger MA, Guendel H. Psychosomatic consultation in the workplace: Do we reach different users by changing the context? BMC Health Services Research. 2014;**14**(Suppl 2):P105

Section 5

Chronobiology of the Respiratory System

Chapter 6

Integration of Chronobiological Concepts for NSCLC Management

Christian Focan, Anne-Catherine Davin, Maryam Bourhaba and Marie-Pascale Graas

Abstract

The authors reviewed pertinent experimental and clinical data allowing to consider the interest of taking into account the temporal dimension ('circadian') for prevention and management of the majority of cancers, i.e., non-small cell lung carcinoma (NSCLC). The universal importance of circadian rhythms has been acknowledged in animal or human situations regarding carcinogenesis and cancer promotion; cell kinetics, apoptosis, molecular genetics, as well as DNA repair mechanisms, platinum resistance...; molecular targets (i.e., epidermal growth factor reception-EGFR); and all lymphoid and immunology machinery components. Also chronotolerance to all chemotherapeutic agents useful for treating human lung cancer has also been evidenced. A few randomized clinical chronotherapy trials were performed in human NSCLC. One limited trial has shown apparent chronoefficiency, while in another one, chronotolerance to 5-fluorouracil and a platinum derivative were confirmed. The limited improvement of outcome in human NSCLC, even through the use of targeted and biological therapies (such as tyrosine-kinase (TKI) or vascular-endothelial-growth-factor (VEGFR) inhibitors; immunotherapy), allows to consider launching specific trials in human NSCLC aiming at either restoring a normal circadian structure of the host or taking into account circadian variations of specific targets. By now unfortunately, no targeted or immunotherapy trials have been launched considering temporal dimension.

Keywords: circadian rhythms NSCLC review

1. Introduction

1.1 Circadian timing system

Life is structured in space but also in time. Biological rhythms have been documented in all processes involved in the malignant transformation of cells as well as in the cellular proliferation of both healthy and tumor tissues [1–5]. All physiological functions expressed their metabolic or specific activities according to a circadian variation [1–5]. This is the case not only for actively dividing tissues but also for all other tissues, such as the myocardium, central nervous system, or organs involved in the metabolization, detoxification and excretion of drugs (kidney, liver) [3–5].

Recent advances identify critical molecular events that rhythmically control drug metabolism and detoxification, cell cycle, molecular targets, deoxyribonucleic acid (DNA) repair, apoptosis, and angiogenesis [3–5]. The coordination of these processes along the 24-h period is ensured by the circadian timing system (CTS) whose hierarchical organization determines chronotherapeutic effects [3–5]. The CTS coordinates physiology and cellular functions over a 24-h period (**Figures 1** and **2**). This circadian physiology is generated or controlled by a central pacemaker, the suprachiasmatic nuclei (SCN) in the hypothalamus. The SCN generate circadian physiology through diffusible signals, including transforming growth factor-alpha (TGF-alpha), epidermal growth factor (EGF), prokineticin-2, cardiotrophin-like cytokine, and neuroanatomic sympathetic and parasympathetic pathways [1–8].

A dozen specific clock genes constitute the core of the molecular clock in mammals [3–6]. These genes are involved in transcriptional and posttranscriptional activation and inhibition regulatory loops that result in the generation of the circadian oscillation in all physiological systems and individual mammalian cells [3–5]. In particular, the circadian locomotor output cycles kaput-brain and muscle ARNT-like protein-1 (CLOCK-BMAL1) or NPAS2-BMAL1 protein dimers play a key role in the molecular clock through the activation of transcriptional clock genes period's (Per's), cryptochrome (Cry's), and Reverb's [3–5, 9] (**Figures 1** and **2**).

Proper circadian regulation is essential for the well-being of the organism, and disruption of circadian rhythms is associated with pathological conditions including cancer [1, 5, 10, 11]. In mammals, the core clock genes, Per1 and Per2, are key regulators of circadian rhythms in central clock, in the hypothalamus, and in peripheral tissues [9–13]. Recent findings revealed molecular links between Per

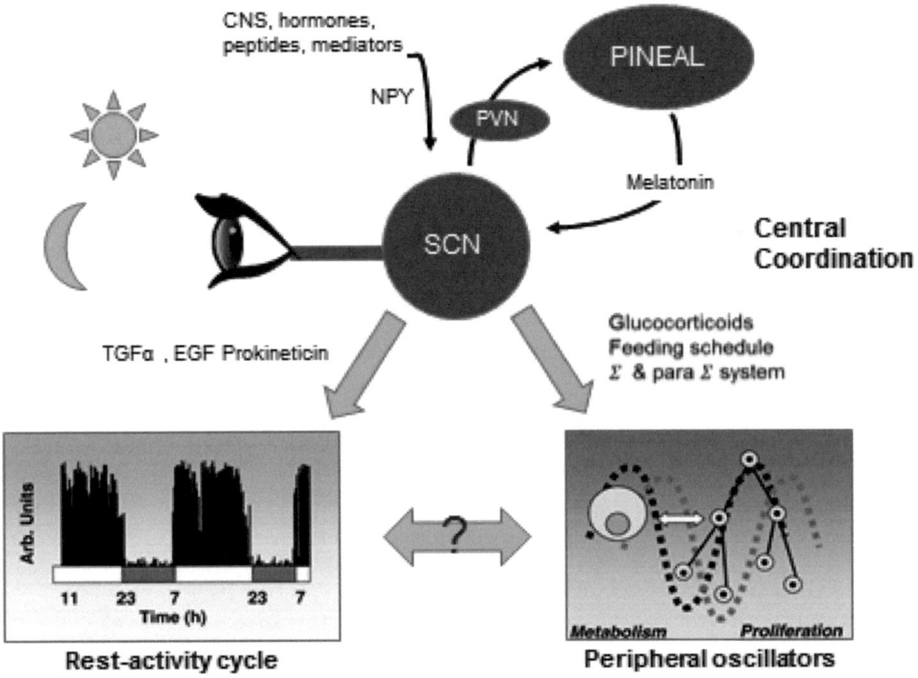

Figure 1.
Schematic view of the circadian timing system (CTS). The suprachiasmatic nucleus (SCN) is a biological clock located at the floor of the hypothalamus. Its period (cycle duration) is calibrated by the alternation of light (L) and darkness (D) through the rhythmic melatonin secretion by the pineal gland. The SCN controls or coordinates circadian rhythms in the body. Abbreviations: PVN, paraventricular nucleus; NPY, neuropeptide Y; TGF-alpha, transforming growth factor α; EGF, epidermal growth factor; Σ, sympathetic (after Levi et al. [3]; adapted).

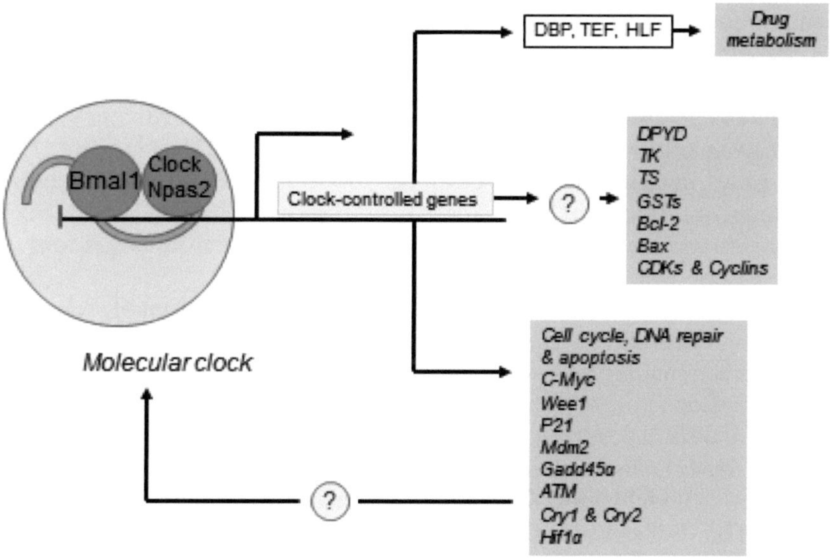

Figure 2.
Schematic representation of the molecular clock and the pathways involved into the control of relevant drug metabolism, cell cycle, DNA repair, and apoptosis in mammalian tissues. The protein dimer BMAL1-CLOCK or BMAL1-NPAS2 (a CLOCK homolog) plays an essential role in the rhythmic transcription of clock-controlled genes. After Levi et al. [3]; modified.

genes and cellular components that control fundamental cellular processes such as cell division and DNA damage [9–13]. New data also shed light on mechanisms by which circadian oscillators operate in peripheral organs to influence tissue-dependent metabolic and hormonal pathways [4, 5]. Circadian cycles are linked to basic cellular functions, as well as to tissue-specific processes through the control of gene expression and protein interactions. By controlling global networks such as chromatin remolding and protein families, which themselves regulate a broad range of cellular functions, circadian regulation impinges upon almost all major physiological pathways including immunological ones [4, 5].

1.2 Aim of this review

In 2002, we performed an overview of accessible experimental and clinical data allowing to believe in possible improvement in NSCLC management through chronobiological considerations. Here we will update our previous review with experimental and clinical recent contributions considering only circadian rhythmicity [14].

It is to be emphasized that we were unable to find any study on that subject using new biological alternatives such as targeted therapies or immunotherapy approaches.

2. Carcinogenesis

Studies performed by Hashimoto et al. on a murine model with circadian-varying lung tumor induction through timed single- or split-dose irradiation have already been reviewed [14, 15].

Cancer development associated to circadian disturbances both in damaged (target) and undamaged tissues and systems [1, 3–5] has been described some years ago. Experimentally, the importance of deregulation of circadian rhythms before the development of liver cancer in rats exposed to diethyl-nitrosamine, a carcinogen that can also induce lung tumors, was reported by Filipsky et al. [16].

Molecular insights illustrate how dysregulation of circadian rhythms might influence the susceptibility to cancer development and provide further support for the emerging role of circadian genes in tumor suppression [12]. Silencing of tumor suppressor genes, such as the Per1—clock core gene, resulting from epigenetic alterations may occur early in lung cancer tumorigenesis [9, 17].

These observations allow considering Per1 gene as a potential target for chemoprevention.

Epidemiologic studies in human beings have evidenced a probable relationship between altered circadian rhythms and tumorigenesis. A high incidence of cancer has been observed in long-term shift workers such as flight attendants, nurses, or industrial workers [18–20]. Recent studies have also suggested that alterations of sleep quality were susceptible to enhance the risk of various cancers including lung cancers [21, 22]. Disruption of melatonin circadian rhythms (peak at night after dim-lighting) could partially explain such observations [23]. However, a large epidemiologic on thousands of Chinese female textile workers apparently failed to confirm an increased risk of lung carcinoma [24].

On the other hand, sport practice and regular physical activity, which are known to facilitate and maintain circadian general activities, may have an inverse effect, thus minimizing the risk of developing a lung cancer [25].

3. Cell kinetics and molecular biology

3.1 Cell kinetics

Hashimoto et al. recently reported that DNA synthesis activity in the normal lung was low but higher during the night [15]. Also a large number of experimental animal studies document circadian rhythm in cell proliferation in spontaneous or transplanted tumors, growing in ascitic fluid or solid phases [1, 2]. Precisely, Burns et al. studied alterations of DNA synthesis rhythmicity in selected organs of mice (i.e., bone marrow) bearing a transplanted Lewis lung carcinoma (LLC) [26].

Colombo et al. [27] reported day/night differences of spontaneous apoptosis in two different murine tumors, one of these being a lung one, in addition to circadian rhythms of division, peaks of apoptosis matching with mitoses valleys [27].

In human, circadian rhythmicity of cell proliferation has been reported for squamous cell carcinomas of the lung, as those of the skin and cervix [1, 2, 14, 28]. Various mechanisms responsible for the deregulation of the cell cycle and enhanced susceptibility to oncogenesis through activation of cell proliferation and cancer promotion have been identified. For example, in NSCLC, overexpression of cyclin D1, and mutation of p16 leading to a shortened and accelerated G1-phase and permanent phosphorylation (and inactivation) of pRb are known; in addition, mutations of p53 (with further impaired apoptosis) or pRb have been observed both in NSCLC and SCLC [29].

3.2 Molecular biology

3.2.1 Clock genes and circadian regulation

Tissues such as the liver, pituitary, and kidney but also the lung exhibit robust circadian rhythmicity in cultures [3–5]. Circadian timers are important for lung functions; for example, there is a well-documented link between diurnal variations in lung physiology (i.e., airway narrowing and inflammation) and nocturnal asthma [30]. Gibbs et al. have studied the cellular localization of core clock genes in both mouse and human organotypic lung slices [30]; they also established the effects of glucocorticoids on pulmonary clock [30]. They were able to demonstrate a marked circadian rhythm in PER2 expression that is responsive to glucocorticoids. Immunohistochemical techniques were used to localize specific expression of core clock proteins and glucocorticoid receptor on the epithelial cells lining the bronchioles (Clara cells and type II pneumocyte cells) in both mouse and human lung tissues [30]. Selective ablation of Clara cells resulted in the loss of circadian rhythm in lung slices, demonstrating these cells to be critical for maintaining coherent circadian oscillations in the lung tissue. The coexpression of glucocorticoid receptor and core clock components establishes them as a likely interface between humoral suprachiasmatic nucleus output and circadian lung physiology [30].

Clock genes or proteins PER1 and PER2 have been linked to DNA damage response pathways in a series of studies, involving among others Lewis lung carcinoma (LLC) cells [3, 6, 9, 11–13]. Overexpression of either PER1 or PER2 in cancer cells inhibits their neoplastic growth both in vitro and in vivo and increases their apoptotic rate [13]. Also high expression of circadian gene mPer2 is able to diminish radiosensitivity of LLC and EMT6 cells with decreased expression of bax and p53 and increased expression of c-myc and bcl-2 [12, 13, 31]. This type of observations illustrates that the circadian system is involved in the protection and restoration of tumor cells, i.e., those of LC, against environmental detriments, such as gamma irradiation [13]. The gene, mPer2, might be considered as an inhibitor of tumor radiotherapy effects [32].

Downregulation of Per1 or Per2 enhanced tumor growth (i.e., of LLC cells) in vitro [12, 13, 31, 33]. Thus Per1 and Per2 exert their tumor suppressor functions in a circadian time-dependent manner [9, 31–33]. Also downregulation of Per1 or Per2 increases tumor growth only at given specific times of the day [12]. These optimal times may be shifted in tumors that have mutant period genes [12].

Overexpression of Per1 makes human cancer cells sensitive to DNA damage-included apoptosis; in contrast, inhibition of Per1 in similarly treated cells blunted apoptosis [9]. The apoptotic phenotype was associated with altered expression of key cell cycle regulators. In addition, Per1 interacted with the checkpoint proteins ATM and Chk2. Ectopic expression of Per1 in human NSCLC cell lines led to significant growth reduction [6, 9]. Per1 m-RNA expression was high in the normal lung and downregulated in a large panel of tumor samples from NSCLC patient samples as well as in lung cancer cell lines [3–6, 8, 11]. In addition, Gery et al. showed that ectopic or forced expression of Per1 in NSCLC cell lines led to growth inhibition, G2M cell cycle arrest, apoptosis, and reduced clonogenic potential [6, 17]. The influence of Per1 on cell cycle and apoptosis seems to be p53-status independent [5, 13].

Timeless (TIM) a homolog of a drosophila circadian rhythm gene has circadian properties in exploration in mammals [34]. Precisely its expression is enhanced in lung cancer cell lines where its knockdown was related to the induction of apoptosis, suppression of proliferation, and clonogenic growth [34]. In surgically resected specimens from 88 consecutive patients, high TIM protein levels as gauged by immunohistochemistry (IHC) correlated with poor overall survival [34, 35].

Taken together those results support clearly the hypothesis that circadian rhythm disruption plays an important role in lung tumorigenesis, as well as a link between circadian epigenetic regulation and cancer development.

3.2.2 Circadian regulation of tumor blood flow and angiogenesis

Hori et al. working on experimental Sato lung tumor were able to correlate biological time of greatest tumor growth and highest tissue blood flow (during dark span) [36]. This finding strongly suggests that tumor tissue blood flow has a determining influence on tumor proliferative activity and that tumor growth is influenced by circadian variation in tumor tissue blood flow [36].

These results were confirmed by Blumenthal et al. who also showed that the blood flow rhythm may differ between tumor and normal tissues, thus creating a window of opportunity when tumors could be targeted with a therapeutic agent such as vascular endothelial growth factor (VEGF) inhibitors [37].

The molecular mechanism regulating circadian expression of VEGF in tumor cells (Lewis lung carcinoma cells among others) has been investigated by Koyanagi et al. [38]. They found that the expression of VEGF in hypoxic tumor cells was affected by the circadian organization of molecular clockwork. The core circadian oscillator is composed of an autoregulatory transcription-translation feedback loop in which clock and BMAL1 are positive regulators and period (Per) and cryptochrome (Cry) genes whose expression in the implanted tumor cells showed also a circadian oscillation act as negative ones. The levels of VEGF m-ribonucleic acid (RNA) in tumor cells implanted in mice rose substantially in response to hypoxia, but the levels fluctuated rhythmically in a circadian fashion. These findings support the notion that monitoring of circadian rhythm in VEGF production may be useful for choosing the most appropriate time of day (i.e., when VEGF production is increased) for administrating antiangiogenic agents [38].

In order to identify possible mechanisms underlying tumor progression related to circadian disrhythmicity, Yasumina et al. injected epidermoid HeLa cells in nude mice exposed to a 24-h light cycle (L/L) or to a "normal" 12-h light/dark cycle (L/D) [39]. A significant increase in tumor volume in the L/L group compared with the L/D group was observed. In addition, tumor microvessels and stroma were strongly increased in L/L mice but were not associated to an increase in the production of VEGF. DNA microarray analysis showed enhanced expression of WNT10A (wingless gene 10A). WNT10A could stimulate growth of both microvascular endothelial cells and fibroblasts in tumors from light-stressed mice, along with marked increases in angio-/stromagenesis [39]. Thus, WNT10A may be a novel angio-/stromagenic growth factor. These findings also suggest that circadian disruption induces the progression of malignant tumors via a WNT signaling pathway in models involving tumor cells similar to that encountered in human NSCLC [39].

3.2.3 Circadian regulation of epidermal growth factor (EGF) and epidermal growth factor receptor (EGFR) pathways

Binding parameters and constant dissociation of EGFR circadian variations, peaking late in dark span, were related to DNA synthesis activity variations in actively dividing mouse tissues [40]. EGFR by itself was found to be capable of phase shifting the prominent circadian rhythm of DNA synthesis, i.e., in the esophagus [40, 41]. Phosphorylation of the cyclic monophosphate (cAMP) response element-binding protein (CREB) and SER-133-phospho-CREB (PCREB) is a transcriptional factor that may regulate circadian cell rhythmicity [41]. Concentrations of EGF (and nerve growth factor (NGF)) were monitored in mouse saliva [42]; both growth factors exhibited identical diurnal variations, peaking between 12:00 and 20:00 h. Otherwise, the effect of EGF injections on cell kinetics of mouse tongue epithelium appeared to be time-dependent [41, 42].

Of interest, some studies were also performed in humans. Salivary (on the contrary to urinary or plasmatic) EGF level followed an apparent diurnal rhythm related to feed [43]. It was markedly reduced in the case of oral inflammation or head and neck cancer; in those situations, the capacity of oral mucosal defense could therefore be impaired [43].

EGFR is present in the majority of tumor cells in head and neck cancer [43]. Though circadian rhythmicities in cell proliferation and clock genes have been demonstrated in oral mucosal [45] and in related cancers [1, 2], so far, no study has dealt with the search for circadian variability in EGFR expression in squamous cell carcinomas. However, a circadian rhythm in plasmatic EGF level (with an acrophase around 14:20, a peak-to-trough interval of 26% and a superimposed 12-h frequency) has been reported in metastatic breast cancer patients [45].

As stated earlier, the circadian axis comprises a central clock (SCN; paraventricular areas) and a downstream network of hypothalamic relay station that modulates arousal, feeding, and sleeping behavior among others [4, 46] (**Figure 2**).

Communication between the clock and these hypothalamic signaling centers is mediated in part by diffusible substances that include ligands of the EGFR [4–8, 44, 46] (**Figures 1** and **2**). A significant functional role for EGFR in the suprachiasmatic nucleus is suggested by recent findings showing that epidermal growth factor receptor and its ligand TGF-α are highly expressed in the suprachiasmatic nucleus. Also EGFR activation induces behavioral and physiological effects, strengthening the notion that EGFR can modulate suprachiasmatic nucleus neural function and behavior [4–8, 44, 46]. Furthermore, Vadigepalli et al. confirmed that gene expression response to EGFR is circadian time dependent [8]; this response includes several genes encoding different neuropeptide receptors, ion channels, and kinases. In order to hypothesize the transcription factors underlying the EGFR response, different circadian time-dependent gene expression groups were analyzed for enriched transcriptional regulatory elements in the promoters. Results indicate that several transcription factors such as Elk 1 and cAMP-responsive element-binding protein/activating transcription factor family, known to be "input points" to the core clock network, are playing a role. Taken together, these results indicate that EGFR has a circadian time-dependent neuromodulatory function in the suprachiasmatic nucleus [7, 8].

3.2.4 Circadian regulation of immune pathways

Diurnal variation in immune and inflammatory function is evident in the physiology and pathology of animals and humans [47, 48].

Studies highlight the extent to which the molecular clock, most notably the core clock proteins BMAL1, CLOCK, and REV-ERBα, controls fundamental aspects of the immune response [47–49]. Examples include the BMAL1-CLOCK heterodimer-regulating Toll-like receptor 9 (TLR9) expression and repressing expression of the inflammatory monocyte chemokine ligand (CCL2) as well as REV-ERBα suppressing the induction of interleukin-6 (IL-6) [49].

Disruption of the circadian clockwork in macrophages (primary effector cells of the innate immune system) by conditional targeting of a key clock gene (bmal1) removed all temporal gating of endotoxin-induced cytokine response in cultured cells and in vivo. The loss of circadian gating was coincidental with suppressed REV-ERBα expression. This work demonstrates that the macrophage clockwork provides temporal gating of systemic responses to endotoxin and identifies REV-ERBα as the key link between the clock and immune function. REV-ERBα may therefore represent a unique therapeutic target in human inflammatory disease [49].

Also mechanistically, Bmal1 deficiency in macrophages increases pyruvate kinase M2 (PKM2) expression and lactate production, which is required for expression of the immune checkpoint protein PD-L1 (programmed cell death-ligand 1) in a STAT1-dependent manner (signal transducer and activator of transcription 1). Consequently, targeted ablation of PKM2 in myeloid cells or administration of anti-PD-L1-neutralizing antibody or supplementation with recombinant interleukin-7 (IL-7) facilitates microbial clearance, inhibits T cell apoptosis, reduces multiple organ dysfunction, and reduces septic death in Bmal1-deficient mice [47–49].

4. Chronopharmacology of anticancer drugs active against human NSCLC

4.1 Animal data

Circadian variation in pharmacokinetics (PK) has been observed in rodents for all the drugs routinely administered to LC patients, i.e., pyrimidine derivatives, anthracyclines, vinca-alkaloïds (vinorelbine), topoisomerase inhibitors, taxanes, platinum derivatives, gemcitabine, other antimetabolites, etc. [1, 3–5]. These chrono-PK were expressed though circadian-varying metabolization, detoxification, excretion, and also maximal concentration (CMax) or area under the curve (AUC) [1, 3–5].

Chronotolerance has been observed in rodent studies long time ago for any chemotherapy agents routinely used for NSCLC patients [1–5]. As a recent example, best tolerance and chronoefficacy of gemcitabine alone or in combination with cisplatin were observed with best antitumor efficacy when both drugs were given around their least toxic time schedule, respectively, 11 and 15 hours after light onset (HALO) in animal facility [50]. In an older study, Flentje et al. had also documented the circadian chronoefficacy of cyclophosphamide (CPA) in LLC [51].

Chronotolerance to an experimental radioimmunotherapy with 131 I-anti-carcinoembryonic antigen (CEA) IgG was reported [52]. A 30% increase in maximum tolerated dose was possible when the drug was given at the trough of the bone marrow division activity (around 9 HALO) [52].

Clock, as a member of histone acetyltransferases, controls acetylation of histone 4 required for repair of DNA double-strand breaks thanks to several repair genes such as excision repair cross-complementing group 1 (ERCC1) or activator protein 1 (AP1) [6]. Expression of histone acetyltransferase genes is associated with cisplatin resistance [6, 53]. Histone acetyltransferase inhibition (i.e., by vorinostat) may increase carboplatin and paclitaxel activity in NSCLC cells [54]. The acetyl-CoA-binding motive is found in clock and shows sequence similarity with MYST members, i.e., Tip 60. Tip 60 which is overexpressed in human epidermoid cisplatin-resistant cancer cells [53] exerts a control regulation on several genes implicated in DNA repair (i.e., ERCC1 and AP1) [53].

Furthermore, the promoter region of the Tip 60 gene contains several E-boxes, and its expression is regulated by the E-box-binding circadian transcription factor clock! Thus, clock and Tip 60 regulate not only transcription but also DNA repair, through periodic (diurnal) histone acetylation in cell populations that can be found in human NSCLC [53].

Finally, of interest, diurnal-varying pharmacokinetics of erlotinib (a largely used tyrosine kinase inhibitor (TKI) for treating human NSCLC) has been reported both in xenograft-bearing nude mice [55] and in Lewis tumor-bearing mice. [56]. Circadian rhythm plays a critical role in the pharmacokinetics of erlotinib in mice, and the mechanisms may be attributed to gene expression rhythms of drug-metabolizing enzymes in liver tissues [56]. The inhibitory effect of erlotinib on phosphorylation of EGFR, AKT (type of serine/threonine protein kinase, also called protein kinase B), and mitogen-activated protein kinase (MAPK) varies with its administration time. The results indicate that the antitumor effect of erlotinib is more potent when the drug is administered when the activities of EGFR and its downstream factors increase [55, 56].

5. Human beings

In human as well, pharmacokinetics of some major drugs used in NSCLC have been reported to be circadian varying [1–5, 28, 44]. Circadian variation of plasma 5-fluorouracil (5 FU) concentration has been repeatedly observed when the drug is infused for a few days at a constant rate [57, 58]. This was reported when the drug was given either as a single agent or with a platinum derivative [58]. Similarly, plasmatic concentration of vindesine, a semisynthetic vinca-alkaloïd derived from vinblastine, exhibit circadian variation with peak between 9 am and 3 pm, when infused at a constant rate for 48 h [59]. Also the fixation of platinum ion to plasma proteins was shown to be circadian varying with an acrophase during late afternoon [60]. More recent assessment of circadian variability of cisplatin pharmacokinetics confirmed that cisplatin clearance was 1.38- and 1. 22-fold higher for total and unbound drug with administration at 06:00 pm vs. 06:00 am [61].

Host chronotolerance to anticancer drugs used in NSCLC patients has also been observed in clinical practice. Pyrimidine derivatives such as 5 FU are less toxic when infused during nighttime sleep [1, 3–5, 57, 58]. Also platinum derivatives such as cisplatin, carboplatin, and oxaliplatin are better tolerated between 3 and 6 pm while anthracyclines are less toxic in the morning [1, 3–5, 57, 58]. The first reported chronotherapy randomized trial, based on diurnal cell kinetics, treating mostly NSCLC patients, compared a 40-h sequential chemotherapy beginning either at 10 am or at 10 pm [28]. In this study, patients who received the sequential chronotherapy from 10 am experienced significantly greater granulocyte toxicity [14, 28].

Focan et al. also reported on host chronotolerance of 124 chemotherapy-naïve advanced NSCLC patients, receiving randomly etoposide for 3 days either at 6 am

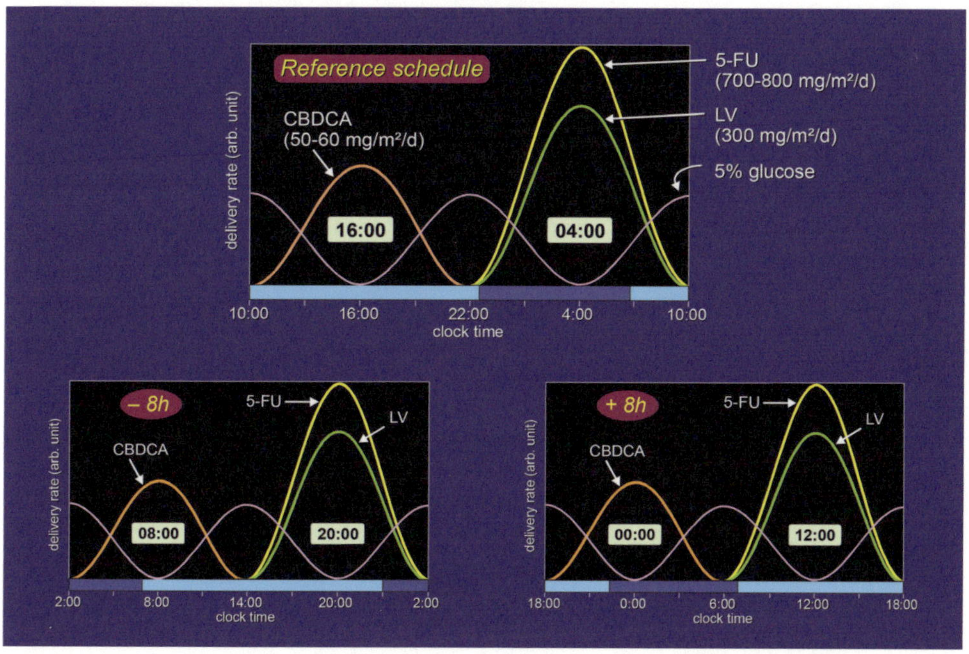

Figure 3.
Programs of ambulatory chronotherapy with 5 FU, folinic acid (leucovorin-LV), and carboplatin (CBDCA). The reference schedule is compared to two others with varying peaks (−8 h; +8 h). Daily delivery is automatically repeated by a chrono-programmable pump (Melodie) five times every 21 days (FFC5_16).

(group A) or 6 pm (group B) and cisplatin at day 4 at 6 pm [62]. A lesser degree of hematological toxicity was documented in group A, while cisplatin was better tolerated in group B [62]. Similar results were reported by Krakowski et al. [63].

Focan et al. also performed a randomized phase I–II trial comparing as first-line treatment, a complex sequential chronotherapy with 5 FU, folinic acid (FOL), and carboplatin with 24-h sinusoidal variation of drug delivery [64] (**Figure 3**). The reference schedule (peaks of 5 FU and FOL at 4 am, peak of carboplatin at 4 pm vs. two other schedules peaking, respectively, at + or – 8 hours, repetition for 5 days every 3 weeks) appeared to be the least toxic one with an overall excellent clinical tolerance [14, 64] (**Figure 4**). Toxicity data were reviewed in order to detect a possible gender effect as had been observed in metastatic colorectal cancer [3–5, 65]. Despite of no significant difference in treatment adaptation or dose intensity between men and women, overall increased serious toxicities were recorded in women versus men. Severe leukopenia and mucositis occurred more than twice as frequently in women than in men (grade 3–4 leukopenia per course, 7.7 vs. 3.2%; grade 3–4 mucositis, 6.6 vs. 1.2%) [14].

According to the results of the phase I–II trial described above [64], a phase II study was further performed on 68 advanced NSCLC previously untreated patients

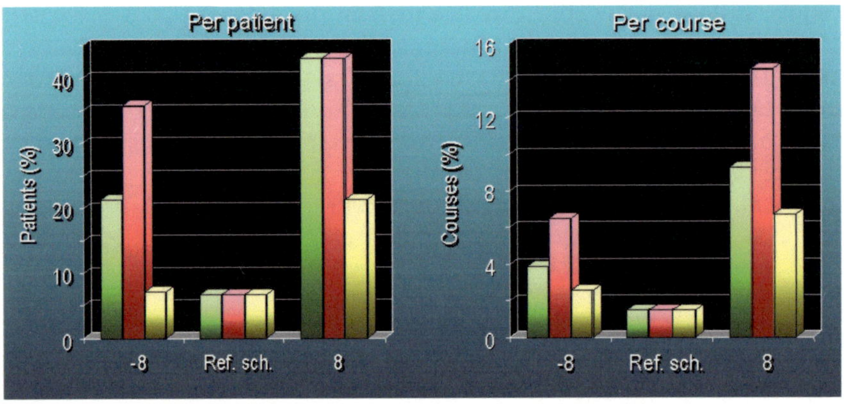

Figure 4.
Tolerability of chronomodulated 5 FU-LV-CBDCA infusion (grades 3–4 toxicities; in green, leucocytes; in red, granulocytes; in yellow, mucositis). Reference schedule was clearly the least toxic one ($p < 0.007$–0.025).

VARIABLE	MALES (275)	FEMALES (84)	p
Hb	10.5	26.2	0.001
WBC	9.8	16.6	0.023
Mucitis	8.3	21.4	0.016

Phase II trial chrono-FFC5_16. Grades 2–4 toxicities according to gender (% courses-p from chi-square)

Table 1.
Gender effect in NSCLC.

with the best circadian schedule [3, 14]. An excellent therapeutic index with a maximum of 17%, grades II–IV toxicities were observed and a gender effect was confirmed (**Table 1**) [3, 14].

Further analyses in advanced colorectal cancers have shown that the pattern of chronotolerance in men was rather sinusoidal with an optimal time corresponding to the reference modality; conversely in women the pattern was damped with optimal peaks of delivery possibly located 6 h later than in men [66]. The male subgroup showed a mean clearance (CL) value twice larger than the value observed in the female subgroup [66]. On the other hand, one has also to remind that the distribution of genes with circadian-varying expression was quite different in men and women in oral mucosa [44].

6. Circadian biological and behavioral determinants in LC patients

6.1 Hormones, immune functions, and tumor markers

A number of groups studied tumor-marker (CEA-carcinoembryonic antigen, alpha-fetoprotein, and others) rhythms but with similar disappointing results [1, 2, 67]. If in controls, a clear group circadian rhythmicity with an afternoon peak around 03:00 pm was evident, in cancer patients, individual variability or absence of rhythm were evidenced [1, 67].

Hormonal, hematological, and rest-activity cycles perhaps might constitute more promising markers of the host's internal circadian time structure. The most prominent hormonal circadian rhythms are cortisol (peak time occurs early in the morning in diurnally active persons) and melatonin (peak time occurs during the first half of the dark period in diurnally active people) [3–5, 67]. Important alterations of the normal circadian profile of these rhythms have been described in lung and other cancer patients with low performance status and high tumor burden [67].

Bartsch and colleagues [68] reported peculiarities in the cortisol and melatonin circadian rhythms in LC patients. Experimental data suggest interactions between interleukin-2 (IL-2; antitumor immune response is an IL-2-dependent phenomenon) and the pineal gland, which also may play a role in the control of immunity and cancer growth [69, 70]. The melatonin rhythm was evaluated in a group of LC patients receiving subcutaneous IL-2 treatment [70]. Prior to IL-2 therapy, none of the patients showed a normal 24-h rhythm of melatonin; IL-2 administration induced a normalization of the melatonin circadian rhythm with a nighttime peak in the majority of cases [70]. This observation suggests that abnormal pineal function in some lung cancer patients might arise in part from altered endogenous IL-2 production [70]. On the other hand, IL-2 administration induced a rise in cortisol with maintenance of 24-h rhythmicity [70].

Melatonin, tryptophan, and 6-sulfatoxymelatonin circadian profiles in blood and urine were compared in 30 advanced NSCLC cancer versus 63 healthy volunteers [66, 71]. All three molecule concentrations were significantly lower in cancer patients with a significant inverse correlation between melatonin and tryptophan levels [71].

Circadian rhythmicity in growth hormone (GH) and insulin-like growth factor-1 (IGF-1) was studied in control subjects and LC patients [72]. GH stimulates IGF-1 production in the liver and other tissues, while IGF-1 can promote cell cycle progression and apoptosis inhibition. GH and IGF-1 also stimulate lymphopoiesis and immune function [72, 73].

In LC patients, a progressive increase in GH and a steady decline of IGF-1 serum levels with loss of circadian rhythmicity were observed. This loss of diurnal rhythms could play a role in carcinogenesis and tumor growth regulation [71–75]. All profiles of time-related neuroendocrine-immune system components seemed to be the advancing stage of disease [71–76].

Mazzocoli et al. assessed altered time neuroendocrine-immune system function in lung cancer patients [75]. Circadian rhythmicity with night acrophases was validated in the control group for hormone serum level (melatonin, TRH, TSH, GH,) and for lymphocyte subset variation (CD3-, CD4-, HLA DR-, CD20-, and CD25-expressing cells). Cortisol, CD6, CD8 bright, CD8 dim, CD16, TcR-delta-1, and delta-TcS1 presented circadian rhythmicity with acrophase in the morning/at noon. In LC patients cortisol, TRH, TSH, and GH serum level and all lymphocyte subsets (except for CD4) showed some altered circadian rhythmicity. Mesor of cortisol, TRH, GH, IL-2, and CD16 was increased, whereas that of TSH, IGF-1, CD8, CD8 bright, TcR-delta-1, and delta-TcS1 was decreased [75]. Peak times however are related similar to those of control subjects [75]. The melatonin/cortisol mean nocturnal level ratio was also decreased in LC patients [75, 76]. Taken together, these results suggested that lung cancer is associated with alteration in the proportions and 24-h profiles of various lymphocyte subsets; this may be related to disease stage and probably altered immune function [73–75, 76].

Lissoni et al. also observed in NSCLC treated by chemotherapy (+/– melatonin) that lymphopenia and altered cortisol rhythmicity were associated with worsened quality of life (QOL), loss of psychosexual identity, and lower spiritual and faith scores [77, 78].

6.2 Host marker rhythms

The persistence of a circadian time structure like that of control normal subjects seems to be an independent prognostic factor, at least in advanced breast or colon cancers [10, 18, 79, 80]. As stated earlier, the strongest circadian rhythms are those of cortisol (with the clinical interest being the morning-afternoon gradient) and melatonin (with a nighttime peak) [2, 4]. Noninvasive easy-to-repeat assessment techniques have been validated for the determination of the 24-h time structure: titrations of cortisol and melatonin in the saliva and 6-hydroxymelatonin sulfate in the urine [81]. Nocturnal urinary 6-sulfatoxymelatonin is also correlated with the proliferation of cell nuclear antigen (PCNA) in lung tumors [68]. Thus, its determination might constitute a noninvasive tool to estimate circadian tumor cell proliferation in lung or other tissues.

Cortisol diurnal rhythm and slope have been related to survival in metastatic breast cancer patients by Sephton et al. [18]. Similarly, the same authors together with Chinese counterparts could also link the quality of persistent diurnal cortisol rhythm to the prognosis (survival) in LC patients [19, 20].

Assessment of the rest-activity circadian cycle by actometry measurements also seems an easy way to estimate the general circadian profile of individuals [1, 4, 5, 82–84]. In advanced colorectal cancer, it was demonstrated in two studies that patients retaining a prominent rest-activity circadian rhythm will enjoy better quality of life and sleep, less fatigue, less depression, and improved survival [82–84]. Such evaluations were proposed to lung cancer patients and validated [82–84]. Focan et al. evaluated rest-activity rhythms in 28 advanced NSCLC before chronotherapy [83]. Better general physical activity and circadian rhythmicity were recorded in those patients receiving also corticosteroids [83]. Hrushesky and his group also studied circadian function in NSCLC patients by actigraphic recordings [82, 84]. They tried to correlate the rest-activity rhythms with sleep disturbances, quality of life (European Organization for Research and Treatment of Cancer (EORTC) Quality of Life Questionnaire (QLQ-C30)) and mood (anxiety; depression—HADS—hospital anxiety and depression scale) [82, 84]. All patients suffered from severe disturbances of daily sleep-activity cycles, but each patient also maintained some degree of circadian organization. QOL measurements were correlated with circadian destructors, fatigue prominent during daytime, and altered moods [82, 84].

Before initiation of their radiotherapy, a high percentage (30–50%) of 185 patients experienced significant disturbances in sleep-wake circadian rhythmicity; these perturbations occurred in both sleep initiation and maintenance [85].

Recent clinical observations have shown that elevated levels of TGF-alpha are associated with fatigue, flattened circadian rhythms, loss of appetite, and depression in patients with metastatic cancer [46]. These data support the hypothesis that a symptom cluster of fatigue, appetite loss, and sleep disruption commonly seen in cancer patients may be related to EGFR ligands released either by the cancer itself or by the host in response to the stress of cancer and suggest that further examination of their role in the production of symptom clustering is warranted [46]. Those observations also suggest to consider the central clock as a possible target for restoration of normal circadian rhythmicity in cancer patients!

7. Clinical trials

7.1 General considerations

During the last decade, the management of NSCLC has evolved [86–97]. Platinum-based chemotherapy remains the standard front-line in treatment of advanced unresectable NSCLC in which cisplatin or carboplatin are combined with another chemotherapeutic agent such as taxanes, pemetrexed, or gemcitabine [87]. However the results in terms of response rate, progression-free survival, and median overall survival remained stable over time [86–97].

Thus, progresses confirmed by phase III trials came from targeted and immunotherapeutic biological approaches. Targeted therapies against EGFR mutations and anaplastic lymphoma kinase (ALK) gene rearrangement have improved the survival in a small proportion of patients whose tumors were expressing these molecular abnormalities [88–91].

Also the recent development and success of immune checkpoint inhibition of programmed cell death 1 (PD-1)/programmed death-ligand 1 (PD-L1) and cytotoxic T-lymphocyte antigen-4 (CTLA-4) for treating metastatic cancers seemed to open a new pavement for fruitful research [86, 92–97].

Unfortunately to the best of our knowledge, despite precise theoretical observations depicted related to circadian expression, on targets of TKI inhibitors, EGFR blockers, antiangiogenic agents, and immune active-agents (lymphoid system; PD1; PDL1), by now no study has been launched to take into account any chronobiological considerations!

8. Chemotherapy

As a matter of fact, in NSCLC, only a few studies deal with considerations on temporal dimension for drug delivery.

Studies from Focan et al. have already been mentioned and reviewed elsewhere [14]. In the first pioneered study [14, 28], a significant better tumor outcome was observed in the group treated at the better dosing time, thus from 10 am for a 40-h sequential schedule [14]. In the second phase III trial using etoposide and cisplatin, despite varying toxicities, there were no differences in overall drug dose intensities nor in tumor outcome gauged by the frequency of tumor responses as well as survival [62]. On the contrary, Krakowski et al. observed an increased dose intensity of drugs when given at their best circadian schedule [63].

According to the results of the phase I-II trial described [59] that had confirmed diurnal tolerance of a complex infusion regimen including 5FU, Fol, and carboplatin for 5 days every 3 weeks, a phase II study was further performed on 68 advanced NSCLC previously untreated patients with the best circadian schedule [3, 14]. Tumor evolution remained within the frame of the literature, but patients enjoyed an improved therapeutic index [3, 14].

Lissoni et al. successively performed small randomized trials (with 20–40 patients per group) in advanced NSCLC patients [67, 68, 77, 78]. They observed progressive improvement of tumor outcome (response rate; 1-year survival, etc.) and quality of life through the association with standard cisplatin-based chemotherapy, melatonin, and sometimes interleukin-2 (IL2) [67, 68, 77, 78]. They have reviewed their results on 370 cases suffering from NSCL and gastrointestinal tract cancers [78]. They confirmed a higher rate of tumor responses and better long-term survival in patients who had received melatonin [78]. These observations were linked to positive circadian effects in cancer-relevant psycho-neuroendocrine and immune pathways [77, 78]. According to these authors, a high degree of faith may positively influence the efficacy of chemotherapy and the clinical evolution of NSCLC by improving the lymphocyte-mediated antitumor immune response and probably general host circadian rhythmicity [78].

Hrushesky's group performed also a randomized blinded trial on 84 advanced NSCLC patients receiving chemotherapy with etoposide and cisplatin together with melatonin or placebo (personal communication). Those patients receiving melatonin during the evening enjoyed higher response rates (29 vs. 8–11%) and longer survival in multivariate analysis (personal communication).

Two meta-analyses appeared to confirm survival benefits associated with melatonin therapy in cancer patients [98, 99]. One analysis has focused upon 8 trials that used a dosage of 20 mg of melatonin, while the second one reviewed 21 clinical trials on solid tumors using various doses of melatonin [98, 99]. Both analyses report that the administration of melatonin reduces the relative risk of death at 1 year by an average of 37%, doubles the frequency of complete response, and reduces the prevalence and/or severity of chemotherapy-induced nausea/vomiting, hypotension, and hematological toxicity. Thus some authors consider melatonin as a probable effective treatment for human NSCLC [100]!

9. Targeted treatments

Despite advances in research and a better understanding of the molecular pathways of NSCLC, few effective therapeutic options are available for most patients with NSCLC without druggable targets, especially for patients with squamous cell NSCLC [86–91].

Chrono-PKs of erlotinib have been investigated in rodents [55, 56]. On the other hand, Iurisci et al. observed an improvement of circadian rest-activity rhythms together with a relief of symptoms in a limited trial on advanced NSCLC patients [101].

Nevertheless, no trial taking into account temporal dimension has been launched at present time.

10. Immunotherapy

Immune checkpoint inhibitors such as anti-cytotoxic T-lymphocyte antigen-4 or anti-programmed death 1 (PD-1) or programmed death-ligand 1 (PD-L1) have induced durable response rates across a broad range of solid tumors. In NSCLC, pembrolizumab and similar antibodies have replaced chemotherapy as first-line treatment for patients with PD-L1 tumor proportion score (TPS) of at least 50% [92–97], while pembrolizumab plus platinum and pemetrexed for those with nonsquamous histology irrespective of PD-L1 expression [92–97].

As discussed in previous chapters, it is conceivable to consider the temporal (diurnal) dimension when administering either targeted or immunologic treatments to lung cancer patients, but, to the best of our knowledge, no study on that subject has been launched to date. We could regret this lack of interest, while dissection of molecular pathways of the circadian clock system has been awarded in 2017 with a Nobel Prize!

11. Radiotherapy

In a single non-randomized limited study, gamma knife radiosurgery for brain metastases of NSCLC was delivered either in the morning (10.00 am to 12:30 pm, 58 cases) or in the afternoon (12:30 pm to 3:00 pm, 39 cases) [102]. Patients treated in the morning enjoyed better tumor local control at 3 months (97 vs. 67%), longer survival (9.5 months vs. 5 months), and a lower rate of central nervous system (CNS)-related cause of death. Those results, which may be related to circadian susceptibility of target cancer cells (? more cells in G2-M phase; more apoptosis in the morning?), prompted the activation of a prospective randomized RTOG study whose results have not yet been published.

With another methodology, Badiyan et al. [103] reevaluated the impact of daytime on tumor outcomes after stereotactic radiosurgery (SRS), in 437 patients NSCLC treated for CNS metastases. They confirmed a cut point of 11:41 am for providing the highest predictive value for overall survival [103].

12. Conclusions

In this review, we have tried to gather pertinent animal and human data supporting the need to take into account temporal dimensions (i.e., circadian) for prevention and treatment of human NSCLC. The importance of biological rhythmicity was evidenced regarding carcinogenesis, molecular biology and genetics, cells kinetics, apoptosis, DNA repair mechanisms, platinum resistance, etc. These observations are fully applicable to human NSCLC.

Some randomized clinical trials for human LC have confirmed chronotolerance and probably chronoefficacy of combined chemotherapy. Furthermore, theoretical considerations allow to propose the application of chronobiological concepts to improve the management of human NSCLC either by working on the host circadian rhythmicity and on circadian variation of targets expression, such EGFR and VEGF receptors, or on the new molecular targets or pathways also circadian varying in their expression (e.g., ERCC1, DNA repair, Tip 60, etc.).

Similarly circadian variations in multiple immunological pathways warrant further interest. These considerations would bring hope to improve overall tumor outcome by optimizing "classical" therapeutic index of chemotherapies but also circadian host rhythmicity by acting on the central clock (i.e., by TKI administration) and/or molecular machinery (receptors, various enzymatic pathways, DNA metabolism and repair, immunology pathways, etc.).

Also the potential role of melatonin as resynchronizing agent and as a potentially active agent warrants further evaluations.

Eventually the increased toxicity of chemotherapy in women is intriguing, peculiarly when host circadian rhythmicity seemed to be implicated.

Acknowledgements

The authors gratefully thank Prof Dr. Francis Levi from Warwick University (UK) for constructive discussions all along the process of this work and for reviews on some chapters. Muriel Focan (Chief Officer Bank of New York, Brussels, Belgium), for reviewing English formulation, and Audrey Stultiens (Clinical Research, Oncology Department, CHC-Liège), for actualizing figures, are also warmly acknowledged.

Conflict of interest

The authors have no conflict of interest to declare.

In homage

To Jeffrey C. Hall, Michael Rosbash, and Michael W. Young who received jointly the Nobel Prize in Physiology or Medicine 2017 "for their discoveries of molecular mechanisms controlling the circadian rhythm."

Author details

Christian Focan*, Anne-Catherine Davin, Maryam Bourhaba and Marie-Pascale Graas
CHC-Liège, ESMO Integrated Center for Oncology and Palliative Care, Oncology Department, Liege, Belgium

*Address all correspondence to: christian.focan@chc.be

References

[1] Focan C. Circadian rhythms and cancer chemotherapy. Pharmacology & Therapeutics. 1995;**67**(1):1-52

[2] Focan C. Marker rhythms for cancer chronotherapy. From laboratory animals to human beings. In Vivo. 1995;**9**:283-298

[3] Levi F, Focan C, Karaboué A, et al. Implications of circadian clocks for the rhythmic delivery of cancer therapeutics. Advanced Drug Delivery Reviews. 2007;**59**(9):1015-1035

[4] Innominato PF, Roche VP, Palesh OG, et al. The circadian timing system in clinical oncology. Annals of Medicine. 2014;**46**(4):191-207. DOI: 10.3109/07853890.2014.916990

[5] Ballesta A, Innominato PF, Dallmann R, Rand DA, Lévi FA. Systems chronotherapeutics. Pharmacological Reviews. 2017;**69**:161-199. DOI: 10.1124/pr.116.013441

[6] Gery S, Koeffler HP. The role of circadian regulation in cancer. Cold Spring Harbor Symposia on Quantitative Biology. 2007;**72**:459-464

[7] Kramer A, Yang FC, Snodgrass P, et al. Regulation of daily locomotor activity and sleep by hypothalamic EGF receptor signalling. Novartis Foundation Symposium. 2003;**253**:250-262

[8] Vadigepalli R, Hao H, Miller GM, Liu H, Schwaber HS. Epidermal growth factor receptor-induced circadian time-dependent gene relation in suprachiasmatic nucleus. Neuroreport. 2008;**18**:1437-1441

[9] Gery S, Komatsu N, Baldiyan L, Yu A, Koo D, Koeffler HP. The circadian gene per1 plays an important role in cell growth and DNA damage control in human cancer cells. Molecular Cell. 2006;**22**:375-382

[10] Davis S, Minck DK. Circadian disruption shift work and the risk of cancer: A summary of the evidence and studies in Seattle. Cancer Causes & Control. 2006;**17**(4):539-545

[11] Chen-Goodspeed M, Lee CC. Tumor suppression and circadian function. Journal of Biological Rhythms. 2007;**22**(4):291-298

[12] Yang X, Wood PA, Ansell C, Hrushesky WJ. Circadian time-dependent tumor suppressor function of period genes. Integrative Cancer Therapies. 2009;**8**(4):309-316

[13] Hua H, Wang Y, Wan C, et al. Circadian gene mPer2 overexpression induces cancer cell apoptosis. Cancer Science. 2006;**97**(7):589-596

[14] Focan C. Chronobiological concepts underlying the chronotherapy of human lung cancer. Chronobiology International. 2002;**19**(1):253-273

[15] Hashimoto N, Endoh D, Kuwabara M, et al. Induction of lung tumors in C3H strain mice after single or fractionated irradiation with X-rays. The Journal of Veterinary Medical Science. 1994;**56**(3):493-498

[16] Filipski Z, Subramabian P, Carriere J, et al. Circadian disruption accelerates liver carcinogenesis in mice. Mutation Research. 2009;**680**(1-2):95-105

[17] Gery S, Komatsu N, Kawamata N, et al. Epigenetic silencing of the candidate tumor suppressor gene Per1 in non-small cell lung cancer. Clinical Cancer Research. 2007;**13**(5):1399-1404

[18] Sephton SE, Sapolsky RM, Kraemer HC, Spiegel D. Diurnal cortisol rhythm as a predictor of breast cancer survival. Journal of the National Cancer Institute. 2000;**92**(12):994-1000

[19] Sephton SE, Lush E, Dedert EA, et al. Diurnal cortisol rhythm as a predictor of lung cancer survival. Brain, Behavior, and Immunity. 2013;**30** (Suppl):S163-S170. DOI: 10.1016/j.bbi.2012.07.019. Epub 2012 Aug 3

[20] Kim KS, Kim YC, Oh IJ, et al. Association of worse prognosis with an aberrant diurnal cortisol rhythm in patients with advanced lung cancer. Chronobiology International. 2012;**29**(8):1109-1120. DOI: 10.3109/07420528.2012.706767. Epub 2012 Aug 13

[21] Chang WP, Lin CC. Relationships of salivary cortisol and melatonin rhythms to sleep quality, emotion, and fatigue levels in patients with newly diagnosed lung cancer. European Journal of Oncology Nursing. 2017;**29**:79-84. DOI: 10.1016/j.ejon.2017.05.008. Epub 2017 Jun 2

[22] Luojus MK, Lehto SM, Tolmunen T, Erkkilä AT, Kauhanen J. Sleep duration and incidence of lung cancer in ageing men. BMC Public Health. 2014;**14**:295. DOI: 10.1186/1471-2458-14-295

[23] Mazzoccoli G, Carughi S, De Cata A, La Viola M, Vendemiale G. Melatonin and cortisol serum levels in lung cancer patients at different stages of disease. Medical Science Monitor. 2005;**11**(6):CR284-CR288. Epub 2005 May 25

[24] Kwon P, Lundin J, Li W, et al. Night shift work and lung cancer risk among female textile workers in Shanghai, China. Journal of Occupational and Environmental Hygiene. 2015;**12**(5):334-341. DOI: 10.1080/15459624.2014.993472

[25] Chen HM, Tsai CM, Wu YC, Lin KC, Lin CC. Effect of walking on circadian rhythms and sleep quality of patients with lung cancer: A randomised controlled trial. British Journal of Cancer. 2016;**115**(11):1304-1312. DOI: 10.1038/bjc.2016.356. Epub 2016 Nov 3

[26] Burns ER, Scheving LE, Tsai TH. Circadian rhythms in DNA synthesis and mitosis in normal mice and mice bearing the Lewis lung carcinoma. European Journal of Cancer. 1979;**15**(2):233-242

[27] Colombo LL, Mazzoni EO, Meiss RP. The time of tumor cell division and death depends on the site of growth. Oncology Reports. 2000;**7**(6):1363-1366

[28] Focan C. Sequential chemotherapy and circadian rhythm in human solid tumours. A randomised trial. Cancer Chemother Pharmacol. 1979;**3**:197-202

[29] Zhang HY, Yang W, Lu JB. Knockdown of GluA2 induces apoptosis in non-small-cell lung cancer A549 cells through the p53 signaling pathway. Oncology Letters. 2017;**14**(1):1005-1010. DOI: 10.3892/ol.2017.6234. Epub 2017 May 24

[30] Gibbs JE, Beesley S, Plumb J, et al. Circadian timing in the lung : A specific role for bronchiolar epithelial cells. Endocrinology. 2009;**150**(1):268-276

[31] Wang YQ, Hua H, Zhu B, et al. The influence of circadian gene mPeriod2 on Lewis cancer cell. Space Medicine & Medical Engineering. 2005;**18**(3):222-223

[32] Zhang J, Zhu B, Liu Y, et al. High expression of circadian gene mPer2 diminishes radiosensitivity of tumor cells. Cancer Biotherapy & Radiopharmaceuticals. 2008;**23**(5):561-570

[33] Chi C, He ZF, Liu Y, Lin XM, Sun CC. Expression and clinical significance of circadian gene Per2 on non-small cell lung cancer (Chinese). Zhuonhua Zhong Liu Za Zhi. 2013;**35**(2):129-131. DOI: 10.370/cma.j.issn.0252-3766

[34] Saez L, Meyer P, Young MW. A PER/TIM/DBT interval timer for Drosophila's circadian clock.

Cold Spring Harbor Symposia on Quantitative Biology. 2007;**72**:69-74. DOI: 10.1101/sqb.2007.72.034

[35] Yoshida K, Sato M, Hase T, et al. TIMELESS is overexpressed in lung cancer and its expression correlates with poor patient survival. Cancer Science. 2013;**104**(2):171-177. DOI: 10.1111/cas.12068. Epub 2013 Jan 7

[36] Hori K, Zhang QH, Li HC, Saito S. Variation of growth rate of a rat tumour during a light-dark cycle: Correlation with circadian fluctuations in tumour blood flow. British Journal of Cancer. 1995;**71**(6):1163-1168

[37] Blumenthal RD, Osorio L, Ochakovskaya R, Ying Z, Goldenberg DM. Regulation of tumour drug delivery by blood flow chronobiology. European Journal of Cancer. 2000;**36**(14):1876-1884

[38] Koyanagi S, Kuramoto Y, Nakagawa H, et al. A molecular mechanism regulating circadian expression of vascular endothelial growth factor in tumor cells. Cancer Research. 2003;**63**:7277-7283

[39] Yasuniwa Y, Izumi H, Wang KY, et al. Circadian disruption accelerates tumor growth and antistromagenesis through a Wnt signaling pathway. PLoS One. 2010;**5**(12):e15330

[40] Scheving LA, Tsai TH, Cornett LE, Feuers RJ, Scheving LE. Circadian variation of epidermal growth factor receptor in mouse liver. The Anatomical Record. 1989;**224**:459-465

[41] Thomson PJ, McGurk M, Potten CS, Walton GM, Appleton DR. Tritiated thymidine and bromodeoxyuridine double-labelling studies on growth factors and oral epithelial proliferation in the mouse. Archives of Oral Biology. 1999;**44**:721-734

[42] Ino M, Ushiro K, Ino C, Yamashita T, Kumazawa T. Kinetics of epidermal growth factor in saliva. Acta Oto-Laryngologica. Supplementum. 1993;**500**:126-130

[43] Christensen ME. The EGF receptor system in head and neck carcinomas and normal tissues. Immunohistochemical and quantitative studies. Danish Medical Bulletin. 1998;**45**(2):121-134

[44] Bjarnason GA, Jordan RC, Wood PA, et al. Circadian expression of clock genes in human oral mucosa and skin: Association with specific cell-cycle phases. American Journal of Pathology. 2001;**158**(5):1793-1801

[45] Haus ED, Dumitriu L, Nicolau GY, Bologa S, Sackett-Lundeen L. Circadian rhythms of basic fibroblast growth factor (bFGF), epidermal growth factor (EGF), insulin-like growth factor-1(IGF-1), insulin-like growth factor binding protein-3 (IGFBP-3), cortisol, and melatonin in women with breast cancer. Chronobiology International. 2001;**18**:709-727

[46] Rich TA. Symptom clusters in cancer patients and their relation to EGFR ligand modulation of the circadian axis. The Journal of Supportive Oncology. 2007;**5**(4):167-174

[47] Deng W, Zhu S, Zeng L, et al. The circadian clock controls immune checkpoint pathway in sepsis. Cell Reports. 2018;**24**(2):366-378. DOI: 10.1016/j.celrep.2018.06.026

[48] Curtis AM, Bellet MM, Sassone-Corsi P, O'Neill LA. Circadian clock proteins and immunity. Immunity. 2014;**40**(2):178-186. DOI: 10.1016/j.immuni.2014.02.002

[49] Gibbs JE, Blaikley J, Beesley S, et al. The nuclear receptor REV-ERBα mediates circadian regulation of innate immunity through selective regulation of inflammatory cytokines. Proceedings of the National Academy of Sciences of the United States of

America. 2012;**109**(2):582-587. DOI: 10.1073/pnas.1106750109. Epub 2011 Dec 19

[50] Li XM, Tanaka K, Sun J, et al. Preclinical relevance of dosing time for the therapeutic index of gemcitabine-cisplatin. British Journal of Cancer. 2005;**92**(9):1684-1689

[51] Flentje M, Akokan G, Reinecke D, Klein HO. Diurnal variations of tumor growth and its influence on cytostatic treatment. Blut. 1981;**43**(2):85-88

[52] Blumenthal RD, Reising A, Lew W, Dunn R, Ying Z, Goldenberg DM Chronotolerance of experimental radioimmunotherapy: Clearance, toxicity and maximal tolerated dose of 131I-anti-carcinoembryonic antigen (CEA) IgG as a function of time of day of dosing in a murine model. European Journal of Cancer. 1999;**35**:815-824

[53] Miyamoto N, Izumi H, Noguchi T, et al. Tip60 is regulated by circadian transcription factor clock and is involved in cisplatin resistance. The Journal of Biological Chemistry. 2008;**283**:18218-18226

[54] Owonikoko TK, Ramalingam SS, Kanterewicz B, Balius TE, Belani CP, Hershberger PA. Vorinostat increases carboplatin and paclitaxel activity in non-small-cell lung cancer cells. International Journal of Cancer. 2010;**126**:743-755

[55] Lin P, An F, Xu X et al. Chronopharmacodynamics and mechanisms of antitumor effect induced by erlotinib in xenograft-bearing nude mice. Biochemical and Biophysical Research Communications. 2015;**460**(2):362-367. DOI: 210.1016/j.bbrc.2015.03.039

[56] Liu J, Wang CY, Ji SG, et al. Chronopharmacokinetics of erlotinib and circadian rhythms of related metabolic enzymes in Lewis tumor-bearing mice. European Journal of Drug Metabolism and Pharmacokinetics. 2016;**41**(5): 627-635. DOI: 10.1007/s13318-015-0284-3

[57] Harris B, Song R, Soong S, Diasio RB. Relationship between dihydropyrimidine dehydrogenase activity and plasma 5-fluorouracil levels: Evidence for circadian variation of plasma drug levels in cancer patients receiving 5-fluorouracil by protracted continuous infusion. Cancer Research. 1990;**50**:197-201

[58] Metzger G, Massari C, Etienne MC, et al. Spontaneous or imposed circadian changes in plasma concentrations of 5-fluorouracil coadministered with folinic acid and oxaliplatin: Relationship with mucosal toxicity in patients with cancer. Clinical Pharmacology and Therapeutics. 1994;**56**(2):190-201

[59] Focan C, Doalto L, Mazy V, et al. 48-hour continuous infusion of vindesine (followed by cisplatin) in advanced lung cancer. Chronopharmacokinetic data and clinical efficacy. Bulletin du Cancer. 1989;**76**(8):909-912

[60] Hecquet B, Meynadier J, Bonneterre J, Adenis L, Demaille A. Time dependency in plasmatic protein binding of cisplatin. Cancer Treatment Reports. 1985;**69**:79-83

[61] Li J, Chen R, Ji M, Zou SL, Zhu LN. Cisplatin-based chronotherapy for advanced non-small cell lung cancer patients: A randomized controlled study and its pharmacokinetics analysis. Cancer Chemotherapy and Pharmacology. 2015;**76**(3):651-655. DOI: 10.1007/s00280-015-280-x

[62] Focan C, Bastens B, Driesschaert P, et al. Circadian tolerance to etoposide and cisplatin as first line treatment for advanced lung carcinoma. Annual

Review of Chronopharmacology. 1990;7:219-222

[63] Krakowski I, Levi F, Mechkouri M, et al. Dose-intensity of etoposide-cisplatin depends upon dosing time. Annual Review of Chronopharmacology. 1988;5:373-376

[64] Focan C, Kreutz F, Moeneclaye N, Focan-Henrard D. Randomised study to evaluate the chronotolerance of a combination infusional chemotherapy with 5-fluorouracil, folinic acid and carboplatin in non small cell lung cancer (NSCLC) patients. Pathologie et Biologie. 2003;**51**(4):204-205

[65] Giacchetti S, Dugué PA, Innominato PF, et al. Sex moderates circadian chemotherapy effects on survival of patients with metastatic colorectal cancer: A meta-analysis. Annals of Oncology. 2012;**23**(12):3110-3116. DOI: 10.1093/annonc/mds148. Epub 2012 Jun 27

[66] Bressolle F, Joulia JM, Pinguet F, et al. Circadian rhythm of 5-fluorouracil population pharmacokinetics in patients with metastatic colorectal cancer. Cancer Chemotherapy and Pharmacology. 1999;**44**(4):295-302

[67] Touitou Y, Focan C. Rhythms in tumor markers. In: Touitou Y, Haus E, editors. Biologic Rhythms in Clinical and Laboratory medicine. Berlin: Springer-Verlag; 1992. pp. 648-657

[68] Bartsch C, Kvetnoy I, Kvetnaia T, et al. Nocturnal urinary 6-sulfatoxy-melatonin and proliferating cell nuclear antigen immunopositive tumor cells show strong positive correlation in patients with gastrointestinal and lung cancer. Journal of Pineal Research. 1997;**23**(2):90-96

[69] Lissoni P. Biochemotherapy with standard chemotherapies plus the pineal hormone melatonin in the treatment of advanced solid neoplasms. Pathologie et Biologie. 2007;**55**:201-204

[70] Viviani S, Bidoli P, Spinazze S, Rovelli F, Lissoni P. Normalization of the light/dark rhythm of melatonin after prolonged subcutaneous administration of Interleukin-2 in advanced small cell lung cancer patients. Journal of Pineal Research. 1992;**12**(3):114-117

[71] Hu S, Shen GHS, Yin S, Xu W, Hu B. Melatonin and tryptophan circadian profiles in patients with advanced non small cell lung cancer. Advances in Therapy. 2009;**26**:886-892

[72] Mazzoccoli G, Sothern RB, Pazienza V, et al. Circadian aspects of growth hormone-insulin-like growth factor axis function in patients with lung cancer. Clinical Lung Cancer. 2012;**13**(1):68-74. DOI: 10-1016/j:cllc;2011.03

[73] Mazzoccoli G, Sothern RB, Parrella P, et al. Comparison of circadian characteristics for cytotoxic lymphocytes subsets in non-small cell lung cancer patients versus controls. Clinical and Experimental Medicine. 2012;**12**(3):181-194. DOI: 10.10087/s10238-011-0153-6

[74] Mazzoccoli G, Pazienza V, Peipoli A, et al. Alteration of hypothalamic-pituitary-thyroid axis function in non-small cell lung cancer patients. Integrative Cancer Therapies. 2012;**11**(4):327-336. DOI: 10.1177/1534735411413269

[75] Mazzoccoli G, Vendemiale G, De Cata A, Carughi S, Tarquini R. Altered time structure of neuro-endocrine-immune system function in lung cancer patients. BMC Cancer. 2010;**10**:314. DOI: 10.1186/1471-2407-10-314

[76] Eismann EA, Lush E, Sephton SE. Circadian effects in cancer-relevant psychoneuroendocrine and immune pathways. Psychoneuroendocrinology. 2010;**35**(7):963-976

[77] Lissoni P, Messina G, Balestra A, et al. Efficacy of cancer chemotherapy

in relation to synchronization of cortisol rhythm, immune status and psychospiritual profile in metastatic non small cell lung cancer. In Vivo. 2008;**22**(2):257-262

[78] Lissoni P, Messina G, Parolini D, et al. A spiritual approach in the treatment of cancer: Relation between faith score and response to chemotherapy in advanced non small cell lung cancer patients. In Vivo. 2008;**22**(5):577-581

[79] Focan C, Levi F, Innominato P. Circadian behaviour of host versus tumour outcome. A review. Pathologie et Biologie. 2007;**55**(3-4):178-180

[80] Innominato PF, Focan C, Gorlia T, et al. Circadian rhythm in rest and activity: A biological correlate of quality of life and a predictor of survival in patients with metastatic colorectal cancer. Cancer Research. 2009;**69**(11):4700-4707. DOI: 10.1158/0008-5472.CAN-08-4747

[81] Nowak R, McMillen IC, Redman J, Short RV. The correlation between serum and salivary melatonin concentrations and urinary 6-hydroxymelatonin sulphate excretion rates: Two non invasive techniques for monitoring human circadian rhythmicity. Clinical Endocrinology. 1987;**27**(4):445-452

[82] Du-Quiton J, Wood PA, Burch JB, et al. Actigraphic assessment of daily sleep-activity pattern abnormalities reflects self-assessed depression and anxiety in outpatients with advanced non-small cell lung cancer. Psychooncology. 2010;**19**(2):180-189

[83] Focan C, Mormont C, Moeneclaye N, Focan-Henrard D, Waterhouse J. Evaluation of rest-activity rhythms in advanced non-small-cell lung cancer (NSCLC) patients. Importance of corticotherapy ? Pathologie et Biologie. 2003;**51**(4):206-207

[84] Grutsch JF, Ferrans C, Wood PA, et al. The association of quality of life with potentially remediable disruptions of circadian sleep/activity rhythms in patients with advanced lung cancer. BMC Cancer. 2011;**11**:193

[85] Miakowski C, Lee K, Dunn L. Sleep-wake circadian activity rhythm parameters and fatigue in oncology patients before the initiation of radiation therapy. Cancer Nursing. 2011. (Epub ahead of print)

[86] Ramalingam SS, Owonikoko TK, Khuri FR. Lung cancer: New biological insights and recent therapeutic advances. CA: A Cancer Journal for Clinicians. 2011;**61**:91-112

[87] Scagliotti G, Brodowicz T, Shepherd FA, et al. Treatment by histology interaction analyses in three phase III trials show superiority of pemetrexed in nonsquamous non small cell lung cancer. Journal of Thoracic Oncology. 2011;**6**(1):64-70

[88] Gridelli C. First-line treatment for advanced non small cell lung cancer harboring activating epidermal growth factor receptor mutation: Epidermal growth factor receptor tyrosine kinase inhibitors or chemotherapy ? Current Opinion in Oncology. 2011;**23**(2): 131-132

[89] Bria E, Milella M, Cuppone F, et al. Outcome of advanced NSCLC patients harboring sensitizing EGFR mutations randomized to EGFR tyrosine kinase inhibitors or chemotherapy as first-line treatment: A meta-analysis. Annals of Oncology. 2011;**22**(10):2277-2285. DOI: 10.1093/annonc/mdq742. Epub 2011 Feb 16

[90] Ceppi P, Papotti M, Scagliotti G. New strategies for targeting the therapy of NSCLC: The role of ERCC1 and TS. Advances in Medical Sciences. 2010;**55**(1):22-25

[91] Ramalingam SS, Maitland ML, Frankel P, et al. Carboplatin and paclitaxel in combination with either vorinostat or placebo for first-line therapy of advanced non small cell lung cancer. Journal of Clinical Oncology. 2010;**28**:56-62

[92] Pauwels P, Remmelink M, Hoton D, et al. PD-L1 testing for non-small cell lung cancer: Belgian guidelines. Belgian Journal of Medical Oncology. 2018;**12**(5):233-238

[93] Zhou Y, Chen C, Zhang X, et al. Immune-checkpoint inhibitor plus chemotherapy versus conventional chemotherapy for first-line treatment in advanced non-small cell lung carcinoma: A systematic review and meta-analysis. Journal for ImmunoTherapy of Cancer. 2018;**6**:155. DOI: 10.1186/s40425-018-0477-9

[94] Assi HI, Kamphorst O, Moukalled NM, Ramalingam SS. Immune checkpoint inhibitors in advanced non-small cell lung cancer. Cancer. 2018;**124**:248-261. DOI: 10.1002/cncr.31105

[95] Lim SW, Ahn MJ. Current status of immune checkpoint inhibitors in treatment of non-small cell lung cancer. The Korean Journal of Internal Medicine. 2019;**34**(1):50-59. DOI: 10.3904/kjim.2018.179. Epub 2018 Sep 3

[96] Bylicki O, Paleiron N, Margery J, et al. Targeting the PD-1/PD-L1 immune checkpoint in EGFR-mutated or ALK-translocated non-small-cell lung cancer. Targeted Oncology. 2017;**12**(5):563-569. DOI: 10.1007/s11523-017-0510-9

[97] El-Osta H, Jafri S. Predictors for clinical benefit of immune checkpoint inhibitors in advanced non-small-cell lung cancer: A meta-analysis. Immunotherapy. 2019;**11**(3):189-199. DOI: 10.2217/imt-2018-0086

[98] Ma Z, Yang Y, Fan C, Han J, et al. Melatonin as a potential anticarcinogen for non-small-cell lung cancer. Oncotarget. 2016;7(29):46768-46784. DOI: 10.18632/oncotarget.8776. Review

[99] Wang Y, Wang P, Zheng X, Du X. Therapeutic strategies of melatonin in cancer patients: A systematic review and meta-analysis. OncoTargets and Therapy. 2018;**11**:7895-7908. DOI: 10.2147/OTT.S174100. eCollection 2018

[100] Zhiqiang M, Yang Y, Chongxi F, et al. Melatonin as a potential anticarcinogen for non-small-cell lung cancer. Oncotarget. 2016;**7**(29):46768-46784

[101] Iurisci I, Rich T, Lévi F, et al. Relief of symptoms after gefitinib is associated with improvement of rest/activity rhythm in advanced lung cancer. Journal of Clinical Oncology. 2007;**25**(16):e17-e19

[102] Rahn DA, Ray DK, Schlesinger DJ, et al. Gamma knife radiosurgery for brain metastasis of non small cell lung cancer: Is there a difference in outcome between morning and afternoon treatment ? Cancer. 2011;**65**(1):414-420

[103] Badiyan SN, Ferraro DJ, Yaddanapudi S, et al. Impact of time of day on outcomes after stereotactic radiosurgery for non-small cell lung cancer brain metastases. Cancer. 2013;**119**(19):3563-3569. DOI: 10.1002/cncr.28237. Epub 2013 Jul 9